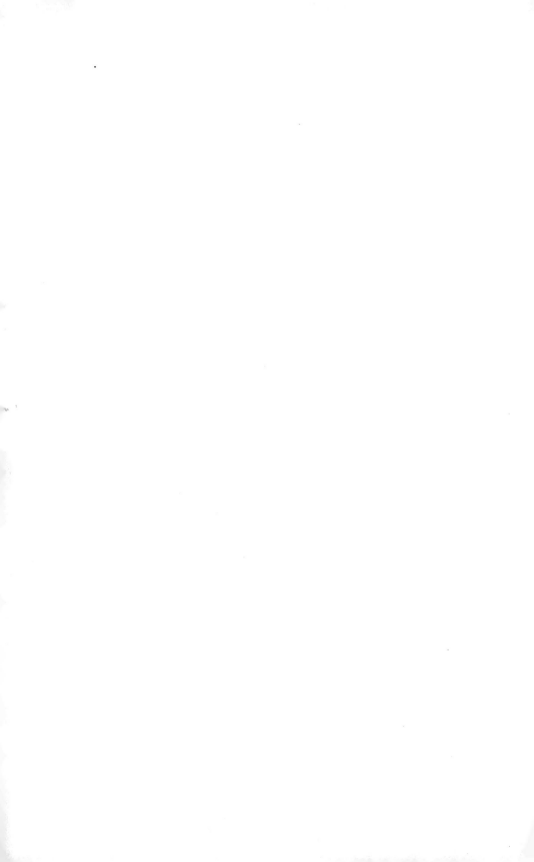

Holistic Dental Care

Holistic Dental Care

Your Mind, Body, and Spirit Guide to Optimal Health and a Beautiful Smile

Stephen A. Lawrence

With David Tabatsky

ROWMAN & LITTLEFIELD
Lanham • Boulder • New York • London

Published by Rowman & Littlefield
A wholly owned subsidiary of The Rowman & Littlefield Publishing Group, Inc.
4501 Forbes Boulevard, Suite 200, Lanham, Maryland 20706
www.rowman.com

Unit A, Whitacre Mews, 26-34 Stannary Street, London SE11 4AB

Illustrations by Flash Rosenberg

British Library Cataloguing in Publication Information Available

Library of Congress Cataloging-in-Publication Data Available

978-1-5381-1397-4 (cloth)
978-1-5381-1398-1 (electronic)

∞™ The paper used in this publication meets the minimum requirements of American National Standard for Information Sciences—Permanence of Paper for Printed Library Materials, ANSI/NISO Z39.48-1992.

Printed in the United States of America

The opinions and information contained in this book are not intended to replace any medical advice or treatment plan, including the diagnosis and removal of fillings and/or root canals, nutritional counseling, and psychological assessments. Any dental treatment should be administered only under the advice and care of a physician or medical team. Whenever appropriate, we encourage readers to seek expert medical help and/or legal advice. This book should be used only as a general guide and not as the ultimate source of information on matters of dentistry, diet, and general health.

The author and publisher shall have neither liability nor responsibility to any person or entity with respect to any loss or damage caused, or alleged to have been caused, directly or indirectly, by the information contained in this book.

With regard to anecdotal scenarios and medical evaluations included in the book, all patient names have been changed or left anonymous.

Relevant scientific data is included as it pertains to a particular subject. Because this book is intended to be a guide and teaching tool for *anyone,* we have attempted to dose out medical information that is manageable and satisfying. Those seeking additional data can reference the bibliography or visit www.wellnessdentalcare.com.

Contents

Acknowledgments   xi

Introduction—*Holistic Dentistry: A Comprehensive Approach
to Health and Wellness*   1

Part I: Our Physical Body   **9**

1   Dental Healthcare 101   11

A Path to Optimal Health and Vitality   12
A Brief History of Cavities and Gum Disease   12
The Three Bs: Bugs, Biofilm, and Balance   14
Dental Disease and Your Health   19
How Long Do You Want to Keep Your Teeth?   21
Great Teeth and Gums   22
What About Flossing?   27
A Word on Electric Toothbrushes   27
Food   28
Tooth Picking, Soft Picks, Oil Pulling, and Diluted Bleach
    Mouth Rinse   33
Six Best Ways to Fight Tooth Decay   38
Caries Management Protocol   41
Adjunctive Therapies   43
Rebuilding the Teeth Naturally   43
Dentistry's Best Kept Secret   44
Rebuilding your Gums Naturally   46
What Can You Do Now?   46

2 **From Our Mind to Our Mouth: Holistic Dentistry and the Medical Health Connection** 49

From Barbers to Bacteria: A Brief History of Dental Healthcare 50
Biology 51
The Discovery of Vitamin C 53
Vitamin C and You 53
Chemistry 59
Dental Fillings and Crowns 60
Metals in Dentistry 61
Root Canal Treated Teeth 61
Anesthetics in Dentistry 62
A Word on Fluoride 64
Chemicals in Dental Hygiene Products 64
Biochemistry 65
Partnering with Your Dentist 65
The Perils of Chronic Inflammation and Oxidative Stress 67
We Are One 67

3 **Nutrition: How "Friendly" Foods Affect Your Teeth and Gums** 69

What Should I Eat? 69
Water 70
Fats, Sugars, and Proteins 71
Essential Amino Acids 73
Vitamins 75
Minerals 77
Essential Vitamins and Minerals 78
Recommended Diets 78
A Deeper Dive into Our Diet 79
Beware the Acid Attack! 80
What About Gluten? 81
Nutrition and Your Immune System 82
Dr. Wright's Recommendations 83
Rebuilding Your Teeth with Good Nutrition 84
Foods and pH Levels and Your Body 85
Final Thoughts 86

4 **Chakras, Meridians, and the Heart: How Matter and Energy Affect Your Oral Health** 89

Physics and the World 90
Quantum Physics 91

Energy Levels and Your Teeth and Gums   96
Kirlian Photography   97
Exploring Chakras   98
Meridian Systems   100
Solutions   100
A Final Thought on Downward Causation   102

Part II: Our Emotional Body   105

5 **Stress Busters: A Roadmap to Inner Peace**   107

The Elephant in Every Room   108
Oral Stress   108
The Big Five   109
From Victim to Victor   115

6 **Love and Wellness**   117

Make Your Own Toothpaste   119
How Your Choices Affect Your Emotional Health   120
The Big Choice   121
Forgiveness   123

7 **The Balance of the Universe and Your Teeth**   125

Practical Tools to Keep Balanced and Healthy   127
Pets as Delegates   127
Play   128
Diet and Nutrition   128
Positive Thinking   129
Prayer and Intention   130
Blessings   130

Part III: Our Spiritual Body   133

8 **Love and Healing**   135

What Is *Dis*-ease?   136
Love Versus Fear   136
The Concept of Free Will   137
Water and Life   137
Free Will Before Birth   138
High and Low Spiritual Frequencies   138
Free Will Protection   139

Your Spiritual Toolkit   139
Protecting Yourself at Home and in Business   140
Everything is Connected   141
Establishing a Spiritual Connection   141
Making the Most of Your Spiritual Toolkit   142

Conclusion   145

Notes   149

Bibliography   157

Index   163

About the Authors   171

Acknowledgments

As a first-time author I am humbled by the hundreds of people, patients, and professionals who have made such a big contribution to the ideas, concepts, theories, and helpful tools that make up this book. I would like to express my deepest gratitude to all those special souls that make an endeavor like this possible.

One of my purposes in life is to take 30 years of dental practice and spiritual counseling and share these exciting tools and helpful products with others in a simple and understandable way. It started with the basic concepts taught at the University of Michigan, School of Dentistry, and continued through many lectures and learning, from organizations like the IAOMT and Price-Pottenger Institute.

Daniel L. Tocchini and his Momentus training introduced me to the concepts of commitment, transformation, and fulfilling your life's purpose. William R. Kellas, PhD, Dr. Wayne W. Dyer, David R. Hawkins, PhD, Bruce H. Lipton, PhD, Dr. Ed F. Group, III and many others showed me the connection between the body, mind, and spirit.

Blessed Tiffany, DD and Father Billy Clark are remarkable souls and dear friends and are responsible for most of the concepts and tools in the spiritual part of the book. Their mission to help others choose love over fear, love yourself and others, and remember you are a child of the Heavenly Father help inspire and heal others and the world.

The writing process took 2 years to condense 30 years of ideas and I would like to acknowledge the valuable assistance of Maureen Betty and David Tabatsky who worked through the proposal process. The book's final editing and form took the remarkable assistance of the talented David Tabatsky to transform the ramblings of this dentist and priest and make a beautiful, easy-to-read, and useful book come to life.

I want to thank the talented Illustrator, Flash Rosenberg, for her beautiful drawings throughout the book, my literary agent, Nancy Rosenfeld, and Suzanne Staszak-Silva and her colleagues at Rowman & Littlefield, for taking a chance on this first-time author.

Finally, I want to thank, Colleen, my beautiful wife and partner in life, for her prayers, support, and love, and my wonderful son, Kyle, who motivates and inspires me to be the best father I can be.

Thank you, Heavenly Father, for giving me the talents, motivation, and good health to explore your beautiful and amazing world and help my dear brothers and sisters to obtain and maintain optimal health.

—Rev. Dr. Stephen A. Lawrence

My thanks to Stephen, a true mensch, for such a lovely experience working together, and who knew lollipops could be so healthy? Thanks to our agent, Nancy Rosenfeld, and to Suzanne Staszak-Silva and her colleagues at Rowman & Littlefield.

—David Tabatsky

Introduction

Holistic Dentistry: A Comprehensive Approach to Health and Wellness

I love the sights and smells of my dental office first thing in the morning. The reception area, with its forest green walls, amethyst carpet and cherry wood furniture, has a faint scent of calming essential oils. My office, adorned with pictures of peaceful pastures and natural waterways, has an inviting aroma of incense still lingering from the previous day. I feel at home here, ready to welcome my patients into a positive atmosphere of wellness.

Whenever I welcome a new patient, for example Mrs. Olsen, who was recently referred by a long-time patient, my assistant escorts her into the examination room and offers her a blanket, a heated herbal neck wrap, and a pillow for her knees.

I wonder what fascinating things I will learn about Mrs. Olsen, what concerns she may have—not just about her teeth but the rest of her health. Our conversation will inevitably lead to the importance of wellness, which I define as a state of complete balance, peace, and love in our physical, emotional, and spiritual body.

It's an exciting time to be a dentist, and we have some fantastic treatment options and products available that can help people achieve optimal health and wellness. It's especially gratifying to be practicing authentic *holistic* dentistry, which depends upon viewing a patient through a broader lens than merely his or her teeth and gums. Through diagnosis and treatment, holistic care always considers a patient's physical, emotional, and spiritual condition, and dental health plays an integral role in each of them.

In my case, as an ordained Christian priest, I am guided by my religious faith, and even though this influence does not have a place in my dental practice I do believe our spiritual lives, whether guided by Christian, Jewish, Muslim, or other beliefs, are vital to our general well-being and reaching optimal health.

So while my time is limited with Mrs. Olsen, you can relax with this book, which endeavors to teach you how to improve the health of your teeth and gums, such as simple habits you can do at home, why sugar and bacteria are not the primary cause of your dental problems, and how to repair your teeth and reverse cavities—*without* a dentist. You will learn about all the new things happening in holistic dentistry today, for example, what we now know about dental bugs, diet, a candy that stops cavity bugs in five minutes, another that cleans your teeth and helps stop gum disease, how to choose the right foods and never have another cavity, gum disease, or crooked teeth, and the vital connection between our teeth and the rest of our body.

Continuing our journey of holistic dentistry and wellness, we will show how gum disease and cavities can cause heart disease, diabetes, obesity, arthritis, respiratory infections, cancer, and many other chronic illnesses. We will reveal the poisons that the FDA allows in toothpaste, the association between dental implants and cancer, and how traditional dental anesthetics, which are poisonous, can be avoided. While we're at it, we'll also explain why flossing is worthless to fight gum disease and cavities.

All of this information is vital to your good dental health, but it must also be considered in the context of achieving and maintaining wellness in our body, mind, and spirit, in balance with each other and the universe. When we establish a state of physical, emotional, and spiritual health, we can find peace and love in our life, which offers each of us the opportunity to share this blessing with others, thereby fulfilling the reason we are here on earth and what we are called to do in this life.

While perfect wellness may be almost impossible to maintain, considering the demands and distractions of our fast-paced modern world, it is the journey we are focused on here, not the destination—to find genuine balance through comprehensive good health, and to share the benefits with our family, friends, and communities.

Unfortunately, the current state of dental practice in America is not always focused on these elements. Instead, the biggest concern on everyone's mind is "Will the insurance company pay?"

The patient is always looking for someone else to cover the cost of his or her treatment and the dentist is always looking to adjust the treatment to what the insurance will pay for. Instead of focusing on the best treatment for the patient, including the root cause of the problem, patients and doctors are concerned with how health is being financed.

This climate has led patients to look for a dentist that accepts their insurance, can do what's needed for the least amount of out-of-pocket expense, and has an office close by. It also helps if the dentist is a nice person, perhaps a fellow church member, and entertaining, too—all while seemingly doing a good job.

One of the most misleading quotes I hear to support this mind set among patients is, "I don't care how much you know, until I know how much you care."

Ouch.

A patient may have no idea that their dentist is okay with using toxic, mercury fillings and dangerous metals in their bodies because he or she is willing to put them in their own teeth, and their family's, too. They perpetuate the myths that mercury and nickel are not poisonous, that fluoride is safe and effective, that titanium implants are okay, and that all you have to do is brush and floss. This is because they personally believe these things to be true *and* because these treatments are covered by insurance plans and are the standard-of-care for most dentists, who must adjust their diagnosis and treatments to meet a series of regulations determined by licensing boards responsible for granting them the right to practice.

As you will soon find out, standards of care are based only on physical, evidence-based dentistry, which has proven to be 95 percent false and misleading.[1] These studies rely on old Newtonian models of physics, and have led to a reactionary state of dentistry, based on carpentry and engineering principles that do not address the genuine root causes of disease and imbalance. Traditional dentists drill holes, extract teeth, fill gaps, screw in implants, build bridges, and replace structures, based only on physical science.

It is not considered politically correct by the American dental establishment to study the dangers of fluoride, root canals, implants, or alternative treatments to oral cancer. These practitioners can only use "reputable" research as a basis for their diagnosis and only commonly recognized treatments in their practice.

Fortunately, holistic dentistry takes the whole person into account when searching for solutions and ways to prevent and correct imbalances in the body, mind, and spirit. But not all practitioners are the same just because they tout a "holistic" approach. Some are becoming aware that there is more to life than the physical body that might affect one's health. Some seek effective preventative techniques in trying to understand the influences that result in cavities and gum disease.

However, most of these dentists still focus solely on the physical world. They use solutions from evidence-based science, remove toxins, preach about a good diet, and rely on obsolete technology, based on a principle of *fear.*

This is partly due to the ongoing support of fear-based treatments of allopathic medicine, which attempts to alleviate a condition by treating the body with it's opposite. For example, we treat a fever by trying to stop a high temperature; we try to eliminate bacteria with antibiotics, and we try to eliminate cancer by cutting or burning it out. All of these "solutions" are based on a *fear* of the condition and getting rid of it as fast as possible, instead of examining why the condition exists in the first place.

Consider the extreme precautions some alternative dentists take to remove mercury fillings, such as wearing protective suits to avoid exposure, while also preaching to their patients about the dangers of RCT, fluoride, nickel, and BPA, using the same techniques that traditional dentists employ—practices they claim to oppose!

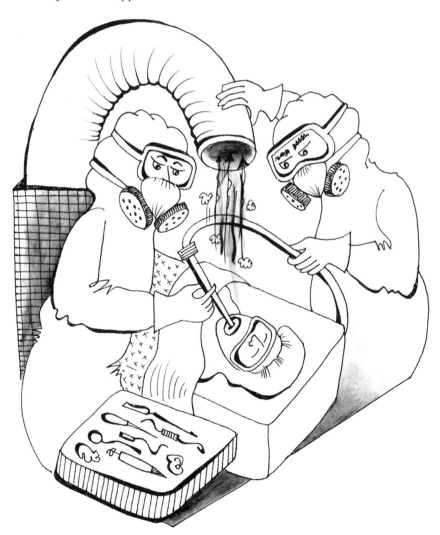

Fear-based dentistry you can avoid

This is mere lip service when it comes to identifying the real root causes of illness and a path to optimal health. These supposedly holistic practitioners do not tell their patients that there could be emotional and spiritual reasons for their dental issues. In fact, it is illegal in the United States for a doctor to even suggest to a patient that their health may be affected by emotional and/ or spiritual causes. As a result, most holistic dentists focus solely on physical, evidence-based practices. But this is not *authentic* holistic dentistry, as it is still based on fear rather than love.

As you will learn in this book, there is a bigger picture when it comes to the way we treat patients, that there is more available to us than physical science.

You can control some of the things required to achieve balance and well-ness, leading to optimal health and vitality. You have a unique opportunity to change what may be necessary to become more at peace in your life and to share love with those around you. We can make this universe a better place by starting with ourselves.

For me, this is driven by the daily practice of my Christian faith, which I will share selectively in the last section of this book. For you, spirituality may come from other sources, but I believe we are all looking for the same thing— to enrich our lives through a commitment to love and gratitude, forgiveness, peace, and a better world.

In this book, I am sharing ideas from a collection of great thinkers, philoso-phers, sacred writings, current science, and some little known truths. Since we are always learning, the process of wellness is constantly changing and evolving as we add new knowledge and expand our awareness.

This began in earnest for me during a biology course at the University of Michigan, when my professor said something I will never forget, which has inspired and guided me in all aspects of my life.

"I have taught you a lot of facts and ideas this semester," he said, "but over the next 20 to 30 years most of that will be proven false. Most of these ideas will be replaced with new ideas and facts, which will be taught to the next generation. You must continue to learn, be open to new ideas, new facts, and new ways of thinking. Always question the present theories, seek truth, and be ready to change your thinking for new truths."

This revelation was powerful and took me a while to fully digest, but once I did, I embarked on a wonderful path of learning and teaching. Since those days, I have witnessed vast changes in science and philosophy.

For example, we used to think that the nucleus of a cell was its "brains," and now we know that is false. We now appreciate the cell membrane's control of a cell and see the nucleus as more of a blueprint for making the structure of a cell.

We also used to think that bugs caused disease and now we know that is false. We will see in chapter 1 how the body's balance and the universe has more to do with causing disease than the bugs around us.

In dentistry, we used to teach patients that plaque caused cavities and gum disease, and that they must brush and floss their teeth or they would lose them. Now we know that is false.

These are just a few examples of what this book explores. By dividing the body (and this book) into three parts—physical, emotional, and spiritual—we will explore wellness from multiple angles, which I believe is the most meaningful way we can improve our lives, including our oral health, specifically our teeth and gums.

Part I—Our Physical Body—is what we are most familiar with, what we can see and touch, and often spend too much of our time mistakenly trying to control. While the body implies our flesh and blood, organs, brain, and so on, this section, while focusing primarily on dental health, will also expand the definition of our physical body beyond the obvious. For example, as we learn about the world of quantum physics, we start to understand that there are parts of our physical body that we cannot see or touch. These are invisible energy fields and patterns that are just as much a part of us as our noses or toes and they can even be measured and controlled. I will introduce some of these concepts and how they relate to holistic dentistry and our general health and vitality.

Part II—Our Emotional Body—explores the connection between our material body, the people around us, and the rest of the world. For example, how do stress, love, hate, fear, pride, influence our health? Fluctuations in all of them affect our immune system, digestion, and hormonal balance. Our habits at work, in play, and during sleep also play a vital role in determining the state of our wellness. For example, we will consider how love heals, how to find love in the ingredients of your toothpaste, why we need to practice forgiveness, and how finding our purpose in life can positively affect our immune system, teeth, and gums.

Part III—Our Spiritual Body—is an elusive concept for some, but may have the most long-term influence on our health and vitality. The free will involved in the choices we make each day—both good and bad—depends on our relationship with the universe and how we define our connection—if we have one—to God and all that comes with that in our lives, including the miracles of healing. This section will explain the effects of water crystals and how they affect us through a practice of love and gratitude. This will also introduce the power of prayer and intention and how it can positively influence our health, because as everyone will learn sooner or later—love *always* wins.

As you may already know and will discover while reading this book, these three aspects of our bodies not only affect each other; they are essentially inseparable, because if one area of the body becomes disrupted, the other two will inevitably suffer, too.

To speak only of one part of our body—for example, our teeth—creates an illusion, because when it comes to total wellness, everything affects everything else. We always take this into account and do our best with the resources we have at our disposal.

This is the essence of the ancient eastern concept of Constant and Never Ending Improvement (CANI). Start wherever you are right now, and you will begin the process of improvement—one small step at a time.

For you or Mrs. Olsen, this journey may begin in the office of a true holistic dentist, where you will experience different services compared to a general dental office. This will vary, depending on the experience, skills, and knowledge of the particular practitioner you are seeing, as each one is a unique individual.

The first visit exam and conversation with Mrs. Olsen will last an hour or more, beginning with a thorough dental and health history, nutritional inquiry, and digital X-rays. I will show her the dental bugs in her mouth, explain the causes of disease, introduce habits she can develop to prevent and repair imbalances, such as thorough dental hygiene instruction, safe and effective teeth and gum care habits, and gentle and effective sonic, hand, and laser treatments for the teeth and gums.

I will show her the tools she has available to restore her optimal health, which include specific testing procedures, such as biocompatibilities to dental materials, heavy metal levels, blood, urine, or stool tests, mineral and nutritional tests, DNA and oxidative stress, EAV, kinesiology, mercury vapor and galvanic testing, among others. Referrals to medical doctors, chiropractors, acupuncturists, psychologists, priests, and other outside practitioners may be made to complete the whole body-focused diagnosis.

I will try to keep it simple, friendly, and not overwhelming, and I'm sure Mrs. Olsen will enjoy some of the routine services we offer, such as aromatherapy and hand and foot massage.

Prevention and a balanced approach to healthy living are the primary focus throughout the patient's diagnosis and treatment, and will continue as a partnership in wellness develops between patient and dentist. When it comes to achieving optimal health and vitality, as well as a beautiful smile, this comprehensive approach offers the best chance for success.

While I always wish I had more time to spend with my patients to fully explain each of these topics, I am so pleased to know that you will have the chance now to use this book as you like to gather useful information and inspiration. Once you've read the first few chapters, you can skip around to different sections, as you search for the steps, ideas, and habits that are most meaningful for you.

I pray that this will be helpful and hope you enjoy our journey together.

—Rev. Dr. Stephen A. Lawrence
Carlsbad, California

Part I

OUR PHYSICAL BODY

We begin by showing you what it takes to keep your physical body balanced and well. It requires that you establish a good diet, maintain a strong immune system, reduce oxidative stress, chronic inflammation, and toxins, increase antioxidants, effectively brush your teeth, irrigate with healthy medications, and using several powerful new tools, which have become the standard form of holistic treatment, designed to keep your teeth and gums healthy and pain-free for a lifetime.

Today's standard of traditional care is based on dated science, which has led to a reactionary state of dentistry that relies on carpentry and engineering principles. Unfortunately, this approach does not address the real root causes of disease and imbalance. Drilling holes, extracting teeth, filling gaps, screwing in implants, building bridges, and replacing structures based only on physical science is *not* holistic dentistry, as it fails to take the whole body into account.

The four chapters you are about to explore will provide a comprehensive foundation of *authentic* holistic healthcare that addresses all of your dental needs while also laying a groundwork for how you can form positive habits in your daily lifestyle.

It is an ever expanding and exciting discovery process to learn more about the body and how we can keep in balance.

1

Dental Healthcare 101

Jack was anxious. All night long, he'd been listening to the howling wind blowing branches from the sycamore tree against his window. By the time the sun came up, Jack felt as if every noise was louder than the one before. But it wasn't a big storm that kept Jack awake during the night. It was the increasing worry inside his head about the pain and discomfort he knew he'd be facing at his dentist appointment that morning. In fact, that dread had left him exhausted and wishing his parents could cancel his appointment.

He rolled over to his bedside table, grabbed a walkie-talkie and flipped it on.

"John, you up?"

Hearing no response from his best friend and next-door neighbor, he tried again.

"John, wake up!"

A few seconds later, Jack heard a familiar voice.

"Yeah, I'm up," said John back, sounding sleepy.

"Hey, see you soon at school," said Jack. "I'll bring a football and we can throw it around at recess."

"Yeah, okay," John said, "but I've got a dentist appointment in the morning and won't get to school until after lunch."

"I've got one too," said Jack, groaning out loud into his walkie-talkie.

John grimaced, pulling his head away.

"That bad, huh?"

"You bet," said Jack. "I can't stand the dentist and his drill."

Really?" said John. "I don't mind the dentist at all or getting a cleaning. Besides, he has lots of prizes to choose from and always gives me a lollipop."

A PATH TO OPTIMAL HEALTH AND VITALITY

While Jack and John have been best friends since they were toddlers, they have been raised in markedly different households. Jack's family eats a standard American diet, snacks on sweets and soda, never brushes or flosses after meals, and relies on toothpastes that do not work at killing bad bugs or supporting healthy gums and teeth. John's family cooks organic fresh foods, drinks raw organic milk, uses effective toothpastes and flossing products, and enjoys cavity-fighting, herbal lollipops and healthy snacks.

John has never had a cavity or problems with his teeth. He doesn't know what a dentist does with a drill and has never had an injection. All John knows is that he gets his teeth cleaned, they feel good afterward, and he gets a cool toy and a lollipop when his appointment is finished. Unfortunately, from an early age Jack has been plagued with cavities, crooked teeth, and vivid memories of long needles, painful drilling, and multiple dental appointments in an uncomfortable chair. To make matters worse, his older sister taunts him mercilessly about how the needles and drilling will hurt, and how he will probably have to have cavities filled and teeth pulled. This always causes Jack a great deal of anxiety while John sees it as just another pleasant trip to a friendly environment.

This story of two similar boys from different families with contrasting cultures, especially regarding diet and lifestyle, demonstrates how healthy habits, especially when instituted at an early age, can shape our dental health and general well-being. It's not only a matter of creating better outcomes for our body. A healthy lifestyle can also reduce unnecessary stress and anxiety, which no child or adult needs to experience, especially when it comes to an upcoming dental appointment.

This is a great time to be a dental patient. We can help stop and/or reverse cavities and gum disease, repair teeth that need treatment with minimally invasive resin fillings, non-toxic porcelains, and zirconia onlays and crowns.

This chapter presents a wealth of healthy habits you can incorporate right away into your daily life so you can have great teeth and pain-free gums like John, while also achieving a lifetime of optimal health and vitality—along with a beautiful smile.

A BRIEF HISTORY OF CAVITIES AND GUM DISEASE

For thousands of years, people rarely experienced dental problems, such as cavities or loss of teeth due to gum disease. People ate local, raw foods, rarely consumed refined or cooked foods, and lived in an environment where few things caused either of these diseases, which are now rampant in many parts of the world.

In fact, archaeological records show that most ancient skulls rarely display any signs of gum disease and cavities. Nowadays, one of the most distinguishing traits of modern skulls is the presence of gum disease, bone recession, and cavities. Two major shifts in the human diet illustrate why we now see more cavities and gum disease than at any time in history.

The first was the development of farming around 10,000 years ago, when much of the world shifted from a hunter-gatherer society to a farming society, which caused a major shift in the oral bacteria in our mouths. Recent research of DNA from tartar on the teeth of skulls from the last 10,000 years shows a dramatic decrease in the diversity in our bacteria, allowing domination by a wide range of cavity and gum disease strains.

The second major shift in our oral bacteria diversity was caused by a much more recent move to eating highly processed flour and sugar.[1]

Both of these shifts have caused major increases in health vulnerabilities in the mouth and the rest of the body and help explain increases in diabetes, heart disease, and other modern day ailments.

Dr. Weston Price and Dr. Pottenger were two of these early researchers in the 1930s and 1940s. Dr. Price, a dentist and researcher, was interested in finding the cause of cavities and gum disease in the current population. Following early research by a contemporary, Dr. Earnest A. Hooten of Harvard University who related these diseases to diet, Dr. Price searched the world, studying the disease rate of various people, looking for a connection between the diets of the people and their instance of cavities and gum disease. He found 14 societies that were free of cavities and gum disease. His health book, *Nutrition and Physical Degeneration*, is a classic nutrition study giving a detailed description of these people, the various diets they ate, and their lack of oral diseases. Many of these societies were isolated from modern diets, had no way of removing deposits from their teeth, had never seen a dentist, and were still free of most diseases.

The research by Drs. Price and Pottenger illustrates the role of diet in the development of our modern-day diseases. The Price-Pottenger Institute, in Lemon Grove, California has become a clearinghouse of information on healthy lifestyle, ecology, sound nutrition, integrated medicine, humane farming and organic gardening. Some of the healthiest families in my practice are avid followers of its resources and training, and like John and his family they are experiencing the benefits of good nutrition.[2]

THE THREE Bs: BUGS, BIOFILM, AND BALANCE

Our bodies are complex and marvelously made. The deficiency of one substance can explain *some* of the changes in our current health status, but we are more complex than this and since none of us have a sterile mouth we must consider a much larger factor in the development of cavities, which is the balance of bacteria in your mouth.

The human mouth has more than 700 different kinds of bacteria and organisms. Most of these bugs, about 660 of them, are good bacteria, one of the first lines of defense of your immune system. These are the probiotic bacteria that are getting so much press lately. They keep us healthy by starting our digestion, fighting off bad bugs and yeast, and maintaining the balance of the mouth's pH and homeostasis. You do not want to kill these good bugs.[3]

In fact, you received all of these bugs from other people.

We are born with a sterile mouth and receive our first bacteria from our mother, which begins in the birth process, then through sharing utensils, kissing, and other bodily exposure, when bacteria is implanted in the baby's mouth from the mother. Experiments in DNA testing have proven that a baby usually gets its first cavity bugs from whomever is the primary caregiver of the child in its early years. This also explains why it's so important for a mother to take good care of her teeth and gums before, during, and after the birth of a child, as it plays a big role in the health of the baby's mouth.[4]

Of all the bacteria in your mouth, only four cause most of your cavities, and one, *strep mutans*, starts every cavity. If you are never inoculated with these bacteria or if you have found a way to get rid of these bacteria, which we will tell you later, you can't get a cavity. You will be like John and never experience a dentist drill or injection.[5]

For example, you can give sterile animals unlimited sugar and refined flour grains and they will never get a cavity because there will be no bugs to change the sugars to acid. There are many other dangers from eating lots of sugar but without strep mutans and the other three bugs that make cavities, they will never develop.[6]

Strep mutans are the first colonizers of a cavity, the first bug to make the sticky substance that hangs on to your tooth, and the main one that makes tooth-destroying acid. This is the bug we use most in cavity experiments and one of the keys to understanding how to fight them.

Strep mutans grow into a colony attached to your tooth's undisturbed surface and eventually form a large structure, called *biofilm*, which is like an apartment building where millions of bacteria can grow and destroy that tooth. If left undisturbed they build a complex colony of bad bugs in the pits,

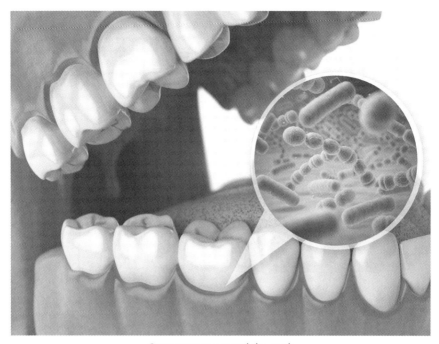

Strep mutans around the teeth
iStock/Bet_Noire

small grooves, and sides of your teeth that are later colonized by the other three acid-loving bad bugs.

All four of these bacteria destroy the enamel of your tooth, demineralizing the surface and creating a *white spot*, which is caused by the dissolving of the enamel's calcium and phosphorous crystal, leaving holes or pores in your tooth.

The bacteria enter your tooth through these holes and live inside it, protected from any cleaning process you normally use. They dissolve the hardest structure in the human body, your tooth enamel, and continue until they are stopped or cleaned out.

This porous surface has a dynamic exchange of calcium and phosphorous from your saliva and nutrition from inside your tooth. The body has a number of ways to repair and rebuild your porous tooth enamel surface *if* the bad bugs can be stopped or killed. Your saliva contains calcium and phosphorous to rebuild and re-mineralize the tooth's enamel and fill in the porous surface if given the right chance.

This reversing and rebuilding goes on between meals and snacks if the body is in balance. The calcium and phosphorous are taken from the saliva

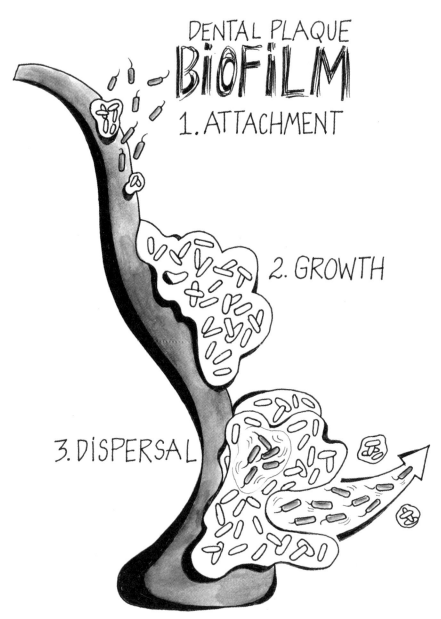

Dental plaque biofilm

CAVITY BALANCE

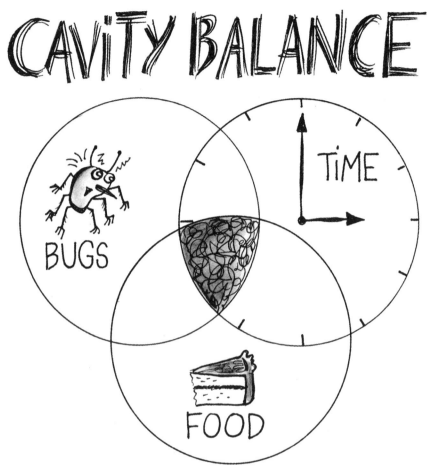

How cavities form

and incorporated into the plaque on your teeth. These minerals fill in the porous holes in the enamel and reverse a cavity. This is why dentists keep reminding patients to not eat between meals and to avoid snacks. The teeth use this time to heal and re-mineralize. Later we will tell you of the phenomenal new products available to the public to effectively kill the bad bugs and rebuild your teeth at home.

We must acknowledge how strong biofilm can be because of the coating that surrounds its structure and how it isolates bacteria from any chemicals or outside influences, such as toothpaste and mouth rinses. These products will just bounce off the surface of the biofilm. This barrier makes the bacteria inside the colony difficult to kill.[7]

This is why some mouth rinses and dental products can be worthless. The barrier protects the bacteria from their effects. Breaking up the colony is vital. This is what your hygienist does with dental tools and microsonic instruments during a professional cleaning. There are now a few products available to the public that can break up the colony and we will introduce them later in the dental hygiene section.

Let's look at how these bugs were initially discovered and how dentists have tried to stop these biofilms from forming. Over the past 150 years the views of dental plaque and bacteria have gone through many changes. The period from the 1800s to 1930s was called the golden age of microbiology. During this time, with the invention of the microscope, researchers singled out specific bugs they thought caused specific diseases.

Dentists studied the plaque of biofilm of the teeth and gums and found various kinds of bacteria, parasites, and organisms. They gave them all names and put them into categories, such as amoebae, spirochetes, streptococcus, Fusiform, and others.

Using the techniques of the time (wet mounts or stained smear microscope sides) scientists identified different groups of disease-causing agents for cavities and gum disease. Dentists identified many oral pathogens in plaque and treatments were tested to kill them. They used dyes, systemic administration of an arsenic-containing antimicrobial preparation, intramuscular injections of mercury, as well as vaccines.

Between 1930 and 1960 dentists came to think that constitutional defects in an individual were more important, that mechanical irritants, such as calculus, overhangs, and the amount of trapped plaque, were the primary causal factors of these diseases.

This ushered in the age of non-specific plaque hypotheses. The belief that there was a specific microorganism that caused a specific disease, such as cavities and gum disease, was replaced by non-specific plaque hypotheses. It was not the *kind* of bug but *how many* of the bugs there were that caused disease.[8]

All plaque was seen as bud bugs. The more plaque someone had on their teeth and gums the more disease they would have. The shift went from the eradication of a specific bug to ways of controlling the amount of bugs. The focus of dental hygiene became stringent plaque control methods of tooth brushing and flossing. Dentists recommended brushing with a stiff toothbrush and daily flossing for patients with dental cleaning twice a year. They thought that if they could completely clean the teeth and gums all day that they could eliminate cavities and gum disease. You will see later why this plaque control belief is so limited and why focusing only on one part of a whole body is doomed to fail.

Some researchers were not convinced in the non-specific plaque hypotheses and their studies showed that flossing was not effective. This research was suppressed and not told to the public because it opposed the current dental plaque theory. But this research indicated that the non-specific plaque hypotheses were not the final answer or the full picture.[9]

The 1960s marked the return to the specific plaque hypotheses, which led to different treatments for specific microbial pathogens and more effective results for stopping cavities and gum disease.[10]

Newer methods of microbial analysis, such as a phase contrast microscopy, scanning electron microscopy, DNA probes, BANA hydrolysis and immuno-assay have transformed today's research.[11]

I have a phase contrast microscope in my dental office. It is the easiest way to quickly test and show a patient the approximately 30 different bugs involved in gum disease. These bugs are big enough and different enough in shape and behavior to be able to name them and tell how many there are and the activity level of the patient's bad bugs. It is an indispensable tool for the dentist and patient to tell the level of disease currently in a patient's mouth and their general risk for further gum and bone damage.

In fact, I would say that it would be difficult for a dentist to know if a patient has active destruction going on in their mouth without a phase contrast microscope examination. A dentist can use expensive, time-consuming DNA testing, but these have difficulty showing some bugs (spirochetes), can't show activity levels on the bugs, number and activity of your white blood cells, or demonstrate visually and vividly the bugs currently in the mouth of the patient.

The present-day Biofilm theory of dental disease is helping us understand the complex behavior and prevention of cavities and gum disease. For example, it helps to learn that biofilms have a protective coating in order to understand why some systemic and locally delivered antimicrobials have not been successful. It also helps explain why some mechanical plaque control and personal hygiene habits continue to be helpful and we can see the importance of getting access to and breaking up the biofilm when trying to prevent and treat gum disease.[12]

Effective tooth brushing, irrigating the gum pockets with antimicrobials, mircosonic cleaning by the hygienist, and low-level laser continue to be helpful but are only a small part of a complex and marvelously made system.

Later, we will address other factors that play a role in the health/disease balance, such as the host's response, emotional and spiritual influences, and ways to stay healthy.

DENTAL DISEASE AND YOUR HEALTH

Let us move on to the systemic theory of dental disease and health. Almost 70 years ago dental researchers found the next piece of the cavity puzzle but were told to keep it quiet and not report it to the public. They were trying to understand how the body rebuilds the teeth and what controls this process. They were investigating how a cavity starts and the imbalances that have to come into play for a cavity to develop.[13]

They found that the first step in a cavity process is not the process of sugar, bacteria, or acid on your teeth. They found that the start to every cavity is the sugar in your gut and resulting imbalance in your organs.

The primary cause of all cavities is not found on the teeth but in the body.

They were trying to understand why the treatments of emphasizing tooth brushing, flossing, and fluoride treatments were continuing to fail and were minimally effective. These modern dental researchers came to understand what holistic dentists have been teaching for years. They are proving that the primary cause of all cavities is an imbalance *inside* the body that controls the nutrient to your teeth.

The body has the capacity to rebuild, repair, and regenerate from a wide variety of disease states. For cavities, the body has a remarkable way to kill bad bugs and rebuild the hydroxyapatite of your teeth. Nutrients coming from the saliva (calcium and phosphorous), nutrients from the inside of the tooth and a vast array of immune system cells fight off invaders and rebuild destroyed tooth structure. It is only when an imbalance occurs to this system and remains long enough that disease forms.

The first step in a cavity developing is an imbalance in your system, specifically in your hypothalamus gland, where a cascade of effects allows a cavity to start. When this gland inside your brain slows down or stops se-creting a hormone that controls your parotid saliva gland, the cavity begins. Without the necessary nutrients the tooth cannot re-mineralize the destroyed tooth structure and the cavity forms. The normal process of rebuilding your teeth between meals and snacks is stopped and the process of acid attacks continues unchecked.

How does the hypothalamus get imbalanced or slow down? We have touched on one of the main causes already, which is too much sugar in the food we eat and swallow. Too much refined sugar in your stomach and system results in an imbalance in your organ—the first steps that result in a cavity. Other causes of hypothalamus imbalance are excessive free radicals exposure (smoking, toxins), lack of antioxidants, not enough fruits and veg-etables, and emotional and spiritual stress.

As we will explore more later, the focus in keeping in balance and in a state of wellness for our dental health is a good diet, strong immune system, reducing oxidative stress and toxins, increase in antioxidants, effective tooth brushing, irrigating with healthy medications, and a few powerful dental aids now available for you to keep healthy teeth and gums for a lifetime.

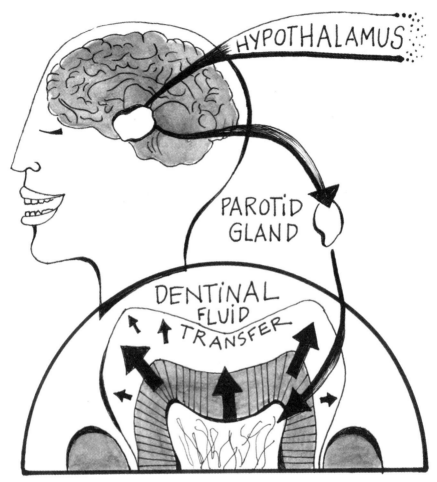

Hypothalamus-Parotid gland endocrine axis

HOW LONG DO YOU WANT TO KEEP YOUR TEETH?

Remember Mrs. Olsen and her first visit to my dental practice? In the introduction I described the anticipation of telling her in a one-hour office visit about her teeth, gums, bugs, diet, and new products available to her. I always regret not having enough time to share everything we know about wellness, some of the fantastic treatment options available, and the connection between our teeth and the rest of the body.

One of the simple questions I ask every new patient during the first visit is, "How long do you want to keep your teeth?" Most patients are surprised and some don't know how to answer it. Some never give me an answer.

It is a leading question, meant to get them to stop and think how committed they are to keeping their teeth. They may begin to wonder if they are doing enough, what they can do better, and if they really want to put the energy into improving how they take care of their teeth and gums *and* achieve general wellness.

The question also allows me to introduce the four things they can do to keep their teeth and gums pain-free for a lifetime. This is summarized in a "Great Teeth & Gums" sheet I offer at the end of the exam, which is included here.

GREAT TEETH AND GUMS

To help keep your teeth and gums for a lifetime you need to do four things:

1. Brush your teeth effectively.
2. Irrigate your teeth and gums thoroughly.
3. Schedule cleanings at the dentist.
4. Strengthen your immune system through good nutrition.

A few thoughts before I explain each step. The list is meant to be short so you will focus on what's most important. Cavities and gum disease start from imbalances in the body and not primarily from bugs or sugar. Researchers have found that brushing and flossing treatment did not stop cavities or gum disease.

I emphasize the first two things on this list because most patients only do two things. Brushing with an effective toothpaste (more on this later) and irrigating with effective antimicrobials are far more effective than brushing and flossing alone.

The third item, cleaning at the dental office, is necessary in this country because of the deep gum pockets and hard calculus that form on a patient's teeth. The hygienist appointment is meant to effectively break up the calculus and biofilm the patient misses, clean out the deep pockets that a patient cannot reach, and reinforce good oral hygiene habits at home. This step is not the most important and most of it can be performed at home if a patient has achieved whole body balance.

The most important step is the fourth—the strength of your immune system and balance of the whole body, which is primarily achieved through good nutrition.

See chapter 3 for more information about nutrition.

All new patients receive an explanation about effective tooth brushing, irrigating with natural medications, the lack of evidence for flossing, and six-month re-care visits. I also offer a treatment plan to address any problems I see. After answering questions and sharing some new trends in dentistry, there is little time left to explain about building up the immune system or how the environment affects their teeth and gums.

This book is meant to explain these steps more fully, especially the fourth one.

Besides describing dental diseases as an imbalance, another way to define cavities and gum diseases is that they are host-mediated bacterial infections. The host (you) mediation is the most important factor. We all have billions and trillions of bugs in and around us every day but our immune system protects us from nearly all of them. The most important factor in health or disease is our terrain—our physical, emotional, and spiritual bodies. Your own whole body keeps the pathogens out, fights pathogens that come in, processes nutrients and immune system cells to fight, and keep the body in balance or homeostasis.[14]

We will start with a fuller explanation of effective tooth brushing and irrigating. Remember that these are easier to explain and for the patient to change but are not the most important steps to optimal health and vitality.

1. Brush Your Teeth Effectively

Brushing your teeth and gums completely cleans all biofilm and plaque you can reach and it should be done immediately after eating or drinking any carbohydrate with an effective antimicrobial toothpaste that kills the bad bacteria, which causes cavities and gum disease.

I teach a circular scrub tooth brushing technique to my patients. This involves taking a soft bristle toothbrush, angling it at 45 degrees to the tooth surface, applying gentle pressure to get some of the bristles under the gums, and rotating the brush in small circles following the curve of the gums.

This is where a lot of bad bugs that cause cavities and gum disease start to form. You are gently brushing all the plaque and bugs that are hiding in this small pocket where the tooth and gum meet. If you use a toothpaste with effective ingredients that kill bad bugs, it will work best when you brush the front *and* back of your teeth.

There are places that the toothbrush cannot clean. The bristles of most toothbrushes cannot clean between the teeth, deep in the gum pockets, in the tooth's top grooves, or around and under dental work. Toothbrushes are made to clean only two of the five surfaces of the teeth—the front and back. This is one reason why tooth brushing alone is not effective at preventing cavities or gum disease. You need the ingredients and other dental hygiene tools to complete the process of keeping your teeth and gums clean.

If you brush like most people, that means up and down and side to side for 30 seconds. This technique misses the biofilm hiding in the crest of the gum pocket and the bacteria between the teeth. When that happens, the plaque biofilm and the bugs double in numbers every five hours and repopulate the teeth and gums.[15]

I tell patients to make a circular pattern on each tooth about eight times and move on to the next tooth. This should be taking at least two to three minutes to complete.

The type of toothbrush you use is not as important as you might think. The first "brushes" were neem tree branch sticks, which were used to clean the teeth much like we would use toothpicks.[16] Today, inside any drug store and many grocery stores you can find hundreds of fancy, complicated toothbrushes. It can be overwhelming to see the number of choices we have to make just to select a manual toothbrush. This includes angled bristles, rotating bristles, short, tall, crisscrossed bristles, color-coded, and musical bristles. The choices seem endless. You can get stressed out just trying to decide on which toothbrush you and your family should use.

I am a simple man. I teach in a simple way. I am sure these different companies all think they are selling the best toothbrush in the world. I am not so convinced. I prefer using a simple soft bristle toothbrush. No fancy gimmicks for me.

I use and recommend the simple Butler GUM toothbrush.

It comes in a few sizes to accommodate different size mouths. This is much better than all the fancy features you will find with hundreds of brands on the market.

I have seen some electric toothbrushes be effective at getting rid of biofilm plaque on the teeth, but most people seem to rely on electric brushes to do all the work and put little effort into effectively cleaning their own teeth and gums.

If you ever wonder where you are coming up short, you can try red dissolving tablets, which you can purchase in a pharmacy, and see the bugs. This uses the same dye as the dentist to reveal the bugs and plaque you are leaving behind. Try this after eating and only flossing. You will see how ineffective flossing is at removing plaque off the teeth and gums.

This leads us to "fake news" and the fallacy of media ads and TV commercials telling us that their toothpaste is preferred because it reduces the plaque on your teeth. These products use pesticides, soaps, and disinfectants to remove the plaque and focus on the old idea that all plaque causes disease. This theory has been proven to be the wrong way to treat disease.

There are many ways to effectively kill *all* the bugs in your mouth. A common way is to rinse with iodine. I have used this in a limited number of patients for specific reasons because an iodine rinse can be effective in completely killing *all* the bugs in someone's mouth and is used to reset the biofilm. For example, for a child with rampant cavities we can reset the bug population of the mouth with a two-minute iodine rinse.[17]

For most of my patients we prefer to kill bad bugs and leave good ones alone. What you need are toothpaste and mouth rinse products that accomplish this. There are many products and ingredients you can find on the market and a dentist like me likes to collect data on these products and ingredients and share them with patients.

You can find many products on the shelves of stores and online, but do they effectively kill the bad bugs and leave the good bugs (and your body) alone? Are they safe for you and your family's health?

Products are always changing, new products appear, new ingredients are used, and the recommended products can change. Any list now may be outdated in a few years.

A toothbrush is not as important as the toothpaste you use, specifically its effective ingredients. I can recommend a few products and companies that currently provide some of the best products in the world.

These include the following products:

Tooth & Gums by Dental Herb Company (www.dentalherb.com)
Dentrarome Plus by Young Living Herb Company (www website)
Closys products by Rowpar Pharmaceuticals (www.closys.com)
PerioBrite by Nature's Answer (www.naturesanswer.com)
Oxyfresh products by Oxyfresh (www.oxyfresh.com)

I am always looking for effective, safe, natural ingredients—free of common toxins and poisons. I have found patients using these products to have the least bad bugs on their microscopic slide tests and less cavities. There may be other effective products currently available and certainly good ones in the future, but this list provides a start.

I test the effectiveness of these products with an expensive strep mutans miscroscope test and a DNA test for gum disease.

I have patients that do not use commercial toothpaste and mouth rinse. They make their own dental healthcare products at home. There are a variety of herbs, essential oils, botanicals, and other ingredients that effectively kill bugs, which we will explain later.

Over the last decade, researchers have tested various products and ingredients to kill specific bugs. If you want to make your own dental products, you can find a list of recommended ingredients in chapter 3.

For example, Dentrarome toothpaste uses an essential oil blend called *Thieves*, which is based on a recipe of oils developed back in the Middle

Ages when the Black Plague was raging across Europe and many people were quarantined away from their homes. When thieves attempted to rob these homes they mixed together a blend of essential oils known to kill bacteria, put them on a cloth rag, and held it over their face so they could enter the vacant homes and steal all the possessions without getting sick.[18]

Various plants around the world contain these essential oils, which also have a special property to kill bad bugs and leave good bugs alone. Thieves is a blend of clove, cinnamon bark, lemon, eucalyptus, and rosemary. These are all powerful oils with amazing properties.

Tooth & Gums is made by the Dental Herb Company, which has put together ancient essential oils and herbs in their toothpaste, mouth rinses, and irrigating solutions. I highly recommend their blog for more information.

If you try to make a mouth rinse for bad breath and gum disease, the ingredients in Dentiva lozenges would be a good way to start. They contain three powerful essential oils—wintergreen, thymol, and eucalyptus.

These and hundreds of other essential oils, herbs, and botanicals have been used for hundreds of years. Many naturopaths, herbalists, DOs, and other alternative practitioners use these and other ingredients to treat patients with bacterial infections, yeast, parasites, and other bodily afflictions.

The Time Factor

The amount of time you allow bad bugs to remain in your teeth and in your gum pockets is crucial to your dental health.

Whenever you eat carbohydrates, the four bugs that cause all cavities use the food you eat to start converting it to acids. They grow a colony called biofilm and multiply on your teeth and in the gum pockets that you miss.

For cavities, the process is almost instantaneous with simple sugars, like sucrose. This sugar is converted to acids and destroys your teeth. This acid attack goes on for as long as you leave the bad bugs alone on your teeth or until your own saliva dilutes the acid chemicals—usually about 20 minutes after you eat simple sugars.[19]

This is why you must brush your teeth thoroughly and as soon as possible after eating a sugary meal or drink!

If you wait too long, it will be too late and the damage will be done. The bad bugs have already changed the sugar to acid and started to destroy your teeth. Brushing for cavity protection *after* the acid attack is worthless.

I see patients all the time who say they brush their teeth twice a day, once in the morning and once before they go to bed. While this regimen can be effective for gum disease, for cavity protection it is nearly useless, and these folks will get cavities unless they perform some other dental disease controls.

Now you might say, well I floss every day. Most people lie to the dentist and hygienist and say they floss every day. Some do, but the vast majority of patients only floss their teeth when they get something caught between their teeth or for fresher breath.

WHAT ABOUT FLOSSING?

Even if you are a daily flosser or floss after every meal or snack, researchers have proven for years that flossing is not as effective as you may think. Yes, flossing gets big particles of food out and can freshen your breath but for cavity prevention and gum disease it is close to worthless.

If you study the effectiveness or lack of it, as it pertains to flossing to get rid of cavity or gum disease bugs, it would get a failing grade. The bugs that cause cavities are in the top grooves of your teeth, in the curves around the contacts of your teeth, and in the small pocket around your teeth. Flossing misses all these bugs.[20]

If you are trying to get big particles of food out of the teeth with floss, this technique still leaves a feast of microscopic food particles around the teeth to feed the bugs for a long time. The bad bugs feast on the sugar and carbohydrates that are still in the saliva, on your teeth, and in the gum pocket for hours and days.

In this case, an oral irrigator is far more effective, as this technique gets rid of the millions of bugs left behind by your toothbrush and floss. I recommend laying down your floss and picking up an oral irrigator with natural antimicrobial ingredients, which will effectively eliminate the rest of the bad bugs.

A WORD ON ELECTRIC TOOTHBRUSHES

Before discussing oral irrigators, I want to address the use of electric toothbrushes and the ever-increasing fancy manual toothbrushes that are flooding the market.

The electric powered toothbrush craze has some good points. The soft bristles heads on these brushes vibrate up to 30,000 times a minute and can effectively break up bug colonies and biofilm on the teeth, around dental work, and even in some gum pockets. They can be especially helpful for patients with manual disabilities, due to illness, age, or lack of hand strength.

But I have found in my practice that most patients are not using these electric toothbrushes effectively. Some push too hard and the bristles slow down or stop. Some move the toothbrush too quickly and miss most of the teeth surfaces and never effectively clean the gum pockets at all. All electric toothbrushes fling off toothpaste in the first few seconds, rendering them less effective when they only dry-brush the teeth and gums.

I love to brush and usually do it for 5 to 15 minutes at a time, usually while I walk around the house, watch TV, work, or do other things. I need to feel the bristles gently going down into the gum pockets just a little. I usually go around the whole mouth twice and even a third time in the lower tongue side of the teeth, which most people miss. I can't do these things with an electric toothbrush so I still use the simple Butler 411 soft bristle model.

FOOD

The last part of our disease formula relates to the food that bugs need to live and grow. You eat food to nourish the body and stay in balance. Your teeth do not need to eat. They have no digestive system and no use for the food you eat. Therefore, keep food off your teeth. Once you finish eating or drinking clean all the food and especially sugar off your teeth, and do it as soon as you possibly can.

We will explore the reason for this in chapter 3 as well as how sugars, carbohydrates, fats, and proteins affect your oral and general health.

2. Irrigate Your Teeth and Gums Thoroughly

Brushing your teeth with healthy toothpaste and a good, simple toothbrush is important but it's not as effective at cleaning bacteria biofilm and keeping your mouth healthy as irrigating. Brushing can help reduce cavities but a toothbrush misses 60 percent of your teeth surfaces and can't effectively clean any deeper than 1 mm under your gum pockets.

Irrigating with an effective liquid is more important than brushing, flossing, and using mouth rinses.

Most people will choose to do two things for their oral health. With this in mind, I emphasize brushing and irrigating. Mouth rinses can be helpful in keeping your breath fresh for a short time. Flossing can get big particles of food out of your teeth and freshen your breath. When it comes to stopping gum disease and controlling bad bugs irrigating is the way to go.

Think of the gum pocket around your teeth like a turtleneck sweater. The rolled-up collar around your teeth is normally one to three millimeters in a healthy person. This pocket is a special place, unlike any other part of your body as it protects the area and special immune system fighters to keep you safe and healthy.

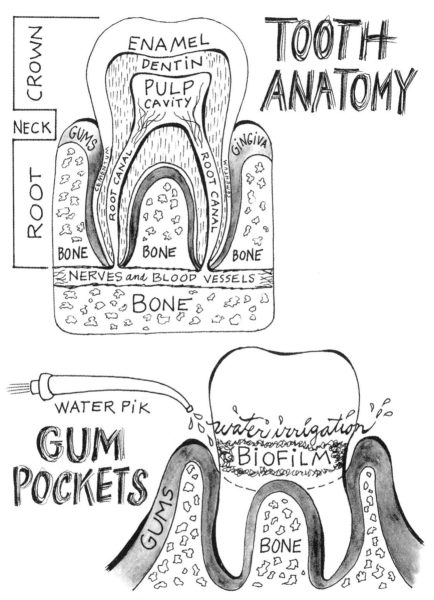

Tooth anatomy and gum pockets

The gum pocket around your teeth is the one place in your body with an open connection between the outside environment and the inside of your body's blood stream. This is the one place that there is no barrier between the outside world full of bugs and toxins and the inside of your body through your blood stream.[21]

Your body has special features in place to protect you and keep you healthy. One of these features is a constant up-flow of fluid from the bottom of the pocket to the mouth. This continuous flow of fluids keeps the movement of bacteria out of the blood stream and up into the mouth. This constant upward flow of fluid can cause problems for the patient or dentist that wants to treat the gum pocket with medications. The upward flow will dilute and expel the medication in only a few minutes. For example, if a patient wants to place toothpaste into the gum pocket or mouth rinse around the gum pocket any product placed into the small pocket will be diluted and expelled by this constant upward flow of fluid.

This is one of the reasons why mouth rinses are not effective in deep gum pockets. The product or medication is pushed out of the pocket and can't remain there long enough to be effective. The flow of fluid is slow but constant and it dilutes and pushes out any toothpaste or mouth rinse from the pocket in 10 to 15 minutes.

Gentle and thorough irrigation is different. The powerful jet flow of water (with medication added in some cases) breaks down the thick biofilm and flushes them out of the pockets. Irrigation can be the most powerful tool you have to clean out your mouth and stay healthy. The idea is to break up the biofilm colony of bad bugs, use a medication to kill the bad bugs, and flush the whole colony out of your gum pockets.

Water irrigator jets can effectively clean up to three millimeters down into your gum pockets. So if you have one to three millimeter gum pockets you can effectively clean your whole mouth with an oral irrigator. The irrigator also washes out big particles of food better than flossing, washes around the areas of the teeth that brushing can't reach and breaks up biofilm colonies better than mouth rinses.[22]

Some of my patients are afraid to Waterpik because they have been told that it just pushes bacteria into the blood. This fear freezes these people into inaction. They stop irrigating and going to the dentist regularly because they are afraid the hygienist will also push bacteria into their blood.

This fear is false and here is why.

A tooth has a pocket that carries up to 500 million bacteria in a pus-forming, bone-destroying colony called biofilm, which forms when a patient does nothing to disturb them.[23] They are hiding from your toothbrush and floss. While untouched, the bad bacteria are a source of chronic inflammation and this infection of bad bugs continues to grow and worsen, spreading to your gum tissue and blood stream, possibly leading to abscessed teeth and gums, tooth mobility, bone destruction, systemic risks of heart disease, lung disease, diabetes, and many other medical conditions we will address later.[24]

You can't get the biofilm with toothbrushing, mouth rinses, or flossing. They double in number every five hours. If you use an irrigator to break up the colonies, kill the bugs with medications, and flush almost all of the 500 million bacteria out of the pocket you risk pushing a few hundred bacteria into the blood stream. It is only a few because your body is made with amazing systems to deal with these bugs. You have many immune system fighters constantly killing the bad bugs in your blood stream, a semi-permeable membrane on your blood vessels protecting the spread of bugs into your body, and a constant up flow of fluid in the pocket reducing the bugs that could invade your blood.

So now you have a healthy gum pocket free of pus-forming, bone-destroying biofilm bacterial colonies, a few hundred bacteria in the blood that are destroyed by the macrophages, neutrophils, and other white blood cells in a healthy person's blood stream.

Leaving biofilm colonies untouched makes no sense. The fear of a small number of bacteria in the blood stream can lead to devastating consequences. The body is an amazing thing and marvelously made. It can handle a few bacteria in the bloodstream, but it can't handle trillions of bacteria, inflammatory toxins, and damage done by unchecked trillions of bugs.

Brush and irrigate thoroughly with effective products that kill the bad bugs and leave the good bugs and your body alone. Your goal is to eradicate the bad bugs, support the healing of your tissues, and strengthen your body's defense system.

3. Schedule Cleanings at the Dentist

If I can clean my teeth and gums with an effective toothpaste and irrigator at home, why do I need to go to the dentist for cleanings? The simple answer is to get the areas you miss and to monitor your health and disease balance.

I recommend you go to the dentist the least amount of times a year that are necessary. If you have 1–3 mm gum pockets, no bleeding or probing, and no bad bugs then a six-month recare appointment is adequate. But how would you know that you only have 1–3 mm gum pockets, no bleeding, and no bad bugs unless a hygienist checks?

If you have pockets 4 mm or deeper, you cannot reach the bottom of the gum pockets to clean out the biofilm colonies. If you have bleeding with occasional tooth brushing or flossing, this is a sign of chronic inflammation. If you start to build up tarter on the teeth you can't clean this at home. You need assistance. How could you know if you have bad bugs unless you're checked with a phase-contrast microscope?

The dentist and hygienist can be your partners in using frequent periodontal gum therapies to eradicate bad bugs, tartar, and infection in your gums before they have a chance to catabolize (eat) your bones and cause many adverse medical conditions.

The important question to ask is: Do I have Gum Disease?

"We are committed to providing you with the best in holistic dental healthcare to keep your teeth and gums and physical body at optimal health and vitality for a lifetime."

This is our oath of care in my office. However, I get some patients who only want their teeth cleaned every six months. They are effectively taking on the dentist's role of diagnosing and forming a treatment plan. I understand that a patient may want to save money (in the short term) or believe that cleanings at the dentist are not that important or they only want the treatment their insurance company will cover.

The infamous six-month recare cleanings, so loved by the insurance companies, dental trade associations, and the media is not based on credible science.

The bad bugs in your mouth double every five hours and build colonies of biofilm in your gums within two weeks, which mature within 90 days. During this time they are well organized, but within three months a mature biofilm colony has formed, which is resistant to your toothpaste and mouth rinse and remains untouched by floss.

By this time, the bad bugs are forming pus, toxins, and chronic inflammatory chemicals and are destroying your bone and tissue and spreading into your blood stream. This damage continues until your six-month recare appointment. Multiply this destruction and infection over a lifetime of six-month cleanings and you can see why you will lose your teeth.

The 6-month recare appointment first became popular when a Howdy Doody TV show recommended to kids that they get their teeth cleaned every 6 months. This period of time was chosen because the tooth powder product advertised on the show generally lasted only 6 months before running out.[25]

It was a good and thoughtful idea because before this time people did not go to the dentist regularly. Dentist visits were usually reserved for toothaches and the treatment was usually extraction. Prevention was rarely thought of and the public could go most of their life without a visit to the dentist. Some people pulled their own teeth when they were painful enough and loose.

Dental researchers have studied the formation of plaque and biofilm in the mouth and found it takes 90 days for dangerous plaque to form. If you have bad bugs (some people don't have any) then a cleaning every 90 days is far more logical, no matter what your insurance company says. If you don't have bad bugs (beware because they are contagious) and have 1 to 3 mm pockets and no bleeding, than you can go 4, 5, or even 6 months or longer. But if you want a partner in your corner, helping you clean where you miss, monitoring your condition, and helping you get better at your own oral hygiene at home, a dentist or hygienist can help.

I have some patients that call the office and tell the receptionist: "All I want is a cleaning." They do this for a number of reasons. Some are trying to save money (in the short term), some hate going to the dentist (imagine that), and some are trying to control all the decisions about their health care.

In America, we are governed by the rule of law. One of these laws states that we cannot treat a patient without first diagnosing them. The patient also cannot bypass the diagnosis of what kind of periodontal disease they have and just start with the treatment.

Another one of these laws states that a patient does not have the expertise to diagnose their own oral health condition. They can decide on what options the dentist offers for their condition but only a dentist can do the diagnosing. They can choose a treatment plan and even refuse treatment, but in America only a doctor can diagnose.

If a dentist allows the patient to diagnose their condition and pick their own treatment plan this will be regarded as unlawful. The dentist may be deemed guilty of malpractice (called supervised neglect).

If you say to your dentist "but all I want is a cleaning" you are asking the dentist to treat you without a diagnosis. In addition to being unethical, he or she would be breaking the law and could lose their dental license.[26]

4. Strengthen Your Immune System Through Good Nutrition

This is where we look at what the body needs to heal and rebuild itself. What ingredients does the body need to rebuild bone? What building blocks does the body need to heal and maintain healthy gums?

The cells of the gums and bone are made from the nutrition you take into your body. The foods you eat and absorb are the ingredients the body needs to build strong gums and bone. We will get into more detail on foods in chapter 3 as well as sharing some of the important ingredients your body needs for healthy gums and bone.

TOOTH PICKING, SOFT PICKS, OIL PULLING, AND DILUTED BLEACH MOUTH RINSE

If I were to add a fifth item to the list of things that can help you keep your teeth and gums for a lifetime it would be tooth picking. I was taught about it

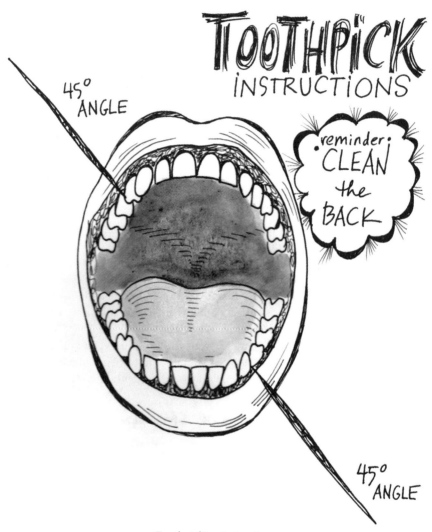

Toothpicking instructions

in dental school and it was re-emphasized to me years later by Dr. Gary Siga-foos, a periodontist I briefly worked for in the San Diego area. He told me that tooth picking is one of the cheapest, easiest, most effective ways to prevent the growth of bacteria in food traps or pockets below the gums. I teach the tooth picking, gentle gum massage technique to my patients with deep pockets and bleeding gums and to get rid of swollen, puffy gum pockets of tissue.

This is a lot like whole body massage, which increases circulation of blood, pushes bad toxic blood out of an area, and allows good oxygenated blood back into the tissues, the gentle massage of deep gum pockets accomplishes the same thing so gums can heal.

A gentle massage of your deep pockets can "shorten" their depth. I have seen one patient go from 12 mm deep pockets to four mm pockets with this technique, which removes plaque from around the teeth that can become tartar and also invigorates the health of the gum tissue.

Toothpicking Instructions

1. Using the side of the tip and not the point, *gently* place toothpick in between the teeth and push in and out ten times.
2. Trace the toothpick along the margin of the gum line. Do this until you have gone in between all of your teeth on the lip (cheek) side.
3. When you are cleaning your lower or upper teeth, aim the toothpick up at a 45-degree angle (as shown).

Note: Always begin in the same area and be sure to rest your hand on your chin or face to help stabilize the toothpick and avoid any slipping.

Perio Aid Instructions

For healthy gums (1–4 mm)

With the aid of a special handle on the Perio Aid you can clean the inside (tongue) surfaces of your teeth (as shown). Follow toothpicking instructions above.

For periodontal pockets (5 mm+)

Keeping the toothpick on the tooth surfaces you can *gently* slide into periodontal pockets. Rubbing in an up and down motion on the tooth surface will remove plaque and bacteria. Do not forget to clean the back surface of your molars.

Soft Picks

The second helpful tool I have been using and recommend is the soft pick. This small, taped, plastic pick has soft bendable bristles on the side. When you move the pick gently between the teeth it scrubs the interproximal surfaces of your teeth and dental work, areas that a toothbrush misses. The toothpick cleans the areas so well that they squeak. It is a very powerful new tool to use to stay healthy.[27]

Oil Pulling

The third tool is *oil pulling*, which has become popular. Many people think it will solve all your teeth and gum problems and can be used instead of brushing and flossing. Many people are jumping on the bandwagon and rinsing daily with coconut oil.

Oil pulling is not new. It has been taught in Ayurvedic medicine for thousands of years. The concept is based on the connection of the mind, body, and spirit. Ayurvedic practitioners teach that all three must be in harmony to promote health. Oil pulling is used to prevent cavities, oral malodor, bleeding gums, cracked lips, and sore throat issues, as well as strengthening the teeth.[28]

But like so many other health techniques, Americans change them to follow their own desires and tastes. For example, I have about a dozen patients in my practice that tell me they faithfully oil pull. Almost all use a nice, pleasant-tasting coconut oil and some do nothing else.

My phase contrast microscope can easily check bug activity. Almost all of the patients that do nothing else have many bad bugs in their mouths and many have worms (parasites) in their gums. None of these oil pullers have healthy bug levels. Why? It's because they have ignored the recommended technique from Ayurvedic medicine, which says you should determine your specific body type and use the appropriate oils. Most of the time the oils are sesame, sunflower, or other oils, but *not* coconut. As you have seen from my list of ingredients for toothpaste there are a few oils (oregano, neem, hemp, and tea tree oils) that have been proven useful for cleansing the mouth of bad bugs.

The technique is to pull or swish 1 to 2 tablespoons of oil in the mouth for 10 to 20 minutes in between the teeth and around the mouth and spit it out. The second step is to brush and floss the teeth and finally swish with a saltwater solution and spit it out.

If you practice the technique as it has been taught with the right oils and proper steps I don't doubt it would be helpful.

Sesame oil has many nutritional benefits with antioxidants of mainly three lignans: sesamol, sesamin, and sesamolin, which have antimicrobial properties and vitamin E. It is thought that these oils lignans act as antioxidants and may act to "clean" the teeth by reacting with the saliva to make a kind of soap. The oil acted on by the salivary alkali and a "soap-making process" known as *saponification* is initiated. During saponification the oil is broken down into droplets and the surface area of the oil is increased. It is believed that the unsaponifiable components of the sesame oil, sesamin, or sesamolin offer protection to the oral cavity because of the antioxidant properties.[29]

Although I don't currently recommend the oil pulling technique because I have not yet seen it work in my practice, it may be useful if done properly.

Dilute Bleach Mouthrinse

The fourth technique that is growing slowly in acceptance with the public is the use of a diluted bleach mouth rinse. Bleach (six percent sodium hypochlorite—NaOCl) is one of the most potent antiseptic and disinfectant agents against bacteria, fungi, and viruses, but it took years before I finally accepted this technique, mainly because bleach does not sound like a healthy product to use in the mouth. I finally went to one of the most trusted proponents of this technique, Dr. Jorgen Slots, a professor at the University of Southern California, and heard his lecture describing the use of a diluted bleach mouth rinse in parts of the world where a safe, effective, and cheap way to take care of their teeth and gums is needed.

The mouth rinse technique was found effective in treating gum disease and cavities in populations that had no access to other ways of caring for their teeth and gums. These people had no money for toothbrushes, irrigation machines, or regular visits to a nearby dentist.[30]

He described the ways neutrophils, macrophages, and monocytes fight off bacteria in the body. Your own immune system cells are using this technique to fight off gum disease and cavity bugs.

The diluted bleach does not evoke allergic reactions, is not a carcinogen or teratogen. It has a century-long safety record in hospitals, animal facilities, and in human drinking water supplies. The ADA Council on Dental Therapeutics has designated diluted sodium hypochlorite as a "mild antiseptic mouthrinse" and suggests its use for direct application to the mouth and around the gums. Diluted sodium hypochlorite has a basic pH, does not risk tooth erosion, and can reduce root sensitivity.[31]

Cheap, safe, effective, and easy to use, a diluted beach mouth rinse is not my first choice but it can be useful, especially for patients that will not irrigate.

Diluted Bleach Mouthrinse Instructions (to be done twice weekly)

1. Place a little less than 2 teaspoons of bleach in 1 cup (8 oz.) of water.
2. Use regular (6 percent) Clorox bleach in the plain blue bottle with the blue cap, with no perfumes or scents, and not concentrated. (For concentrated [8.25 percent] bleach, use 1 teaspoon of bleach to 2/3 cups water.)
3. Mix gently and swish a mouthful of the mixture for 30 seconds.
4. Spit out the extra and avoid rinsing with water for 30 minutes.

Note: You can begin with half of this dose if you need to get used to the flavor.

Instructions for Home Water Irrigation Units (to be done twice weekly)

1. Put 2 teaspoons of bleach in ½ cup (4 oz.) of water.
2. Use as irrigation for the entire mouth, between the teeth, and around the gums.
3. Run plain water through the unit after use to clear out the solution.
4. Avoid rinsing with water for 30 minutes.

SIX BEST WAYS TO FIGHT TOOTH DECAY

Beyond brushing and flossing, which have been used ineffectively for years, there are extremely effective products and foods that you can use to kill bad bugs while leaving good bugs and the rest of your body alone. Here are six I like best.

1. Loloz Lollipops

Many dentists have been frustrated by the fact that children still get cavities. For years, they have hoped for a product that will appeal to children while killing bad bugs and saving good ones. They needed a "smart" bomb that tasted good.

A team of dentists working and collaborating with the UCLA dental school chose a natural antibiotic product and Chinese licorice root extract and combined them with part of the binding sites unique to strep mutans, and they called this new selective product they specifically targeted antimicrobial peptide (STAMPs). They added flavoring and stevia as a sweetener to make a great tasting, anti-cavity lollipop. The lollipop method was first used so that the product would last 5 to 10 minutes before a child chewed up the candy and swallowed it. In that time, the lollipop killed 99 percent of all the bad bugs.[32]

Loloz makes the lollipop in three delicious flavors—orange, berry, and lemon. They also make the candy in lozenge form for those who do not want a lollipop stick showing.

But bugs in the mouth keep multiplying and spreading in your mouth and bloodstream so one lollipop will not kill all the bad bugs. The protocol to effectively lower the number of bad bugs in your whole body is two lollipops a day, one in the morning and one in the evening, for 10 consecutive days. This will effectively lower the number of bad bugs to almost zero and let your body win the cavity fight.

Because strep mutans are contagious, meaning family members, close contacts, and significant others can pass them through food and water, you need to do the 10-day lollipop protocol periodically in order to keep the strep mutans from re-infecting you. I recommend using the protocol twice a year for most people and four times a year for patients at high risk, which includes those vulnerable to cavities, those with an inability to effectively clean their teeth due to a disability, diabetes, or other conditions.

2. Dentiva

It would be nice to have a product for gum disease like this lollipop especially when you can't brush soon after eating. One company began working on this problem and came up with a very good product that does most of what we want a gum disease-fighting product to do. Nuvora has a lozenge that you can dissolve in the mouth that effectively kills most of bad bugs and leaves good bugs alone. It works by dissolving the plaque off your teeth, killing gum disease bugs, and alkylanizing the pH of your mouth.

It is called Dentiva and is a slowly dissolving lozenge with three essential oils—wintergreen, thymol, and eucalyptus, which is a powerful tool you can use to stop the progression of gum disease bacteria and cavity bugs. It is possibly the best product whenever you cannot brush and floss after meals, excellent for after lunch at school or work, and while traveling. Dentiva also has the additional benefit of xylitol use as a sweetener, which greatly influences its antimicrobial power.[33]

3. MI Paste

The third powerful tool is MI paste, a water-based, sugar-free tooth crème that rebuilds your teeth, reverses cavities, reduces sensitivity, and alkalinizes your mouth's pH.

GC America first developed this product to help alleviate tooth sensitivity to bleaching techniques. While they were treating the sensitivity for these bleached teeth, they noticed that some patients with cavities were starting to see them re-mineralize and rebuild. The paste was reversing cavities and making them go away! They found their product, a combination of milk protein, casein phosphopeptide (CCP), and active Ca PO4 (ACP), also had antimicrobial and buffering properties on the plaque, which interfered with the strep mutans and strep sorbinus and repaired the damage these bugs started.[34]

4. Xylitol

The fourth powerful tool comes from birch trees. German chemist Emil Fischer discovered xylitol in 1891. But it wasn't until the early 1960s that it was first employed as a sweetening agent in foods. Since then, it has been widely used in confections, especially in Europe and its popularity among food technologists continues to grow.

In addition to xylitol's sweetening properties, the research of professors Arje Scheinin, Kauko Makinen, and others established that xylitol has measurable inhibiting properties, making it an even more attractive food additive.

Leaf, Inc., a major American manufacturer of confectionary products, recognized xylitol's potential and developed XyliFresh Sugar Free Gum. Leaf is a subsidiary of Huhtamaki Oy, a Finnish conglomerate of consumer goods.

Xylitol products first found success in Norway and Sweden and are now marketed here among dental professionals and health-conscious consumers. Toothpastes, gums, mints, mouth rinses, and candies with xylitol all help wash away cavity bugs and stop them from making acids that eat the tooth surface.

You may be surprised that a dentist would recommend more candy and chewing gum, but hundreds of studies show that the more xylitol gum and candy products you consume the less cavities you will have.[35]

Children who chew two pieces of xylitol gum a day are two times less likely to develop cavities than those that use sorbitol sweetener or sugar-free gum and almost four times less likely than kids who do not chew gum.[36]

Over 150 clinical studies and over 15 years of consumer use abroad prove that xylitol works by helping to reduce plaque acids that can cause decay and by helping to prevent new cavities. Plus, it is a safe and effective adjunct to good oral hygiene and comes in a variety of flavors and products to help improve patient compliance.

Xylitol does not kill bugs like the cavity-fighting lollipops but it is a kinder, gentler way of getting rid of them. Without the sticky glue to hold on and the ability to make acids, the bugs get pushed off the teeth and out of the gums. Over time, it can selectively change the population of bugs in your mouth from bad to good.[37]

This is especially beneficial for expectant mothers.

As you have learned, most kids get contaminated from their mothers with their first cavity-forming bugs. Many research studies have shown that when an expectant mother chews xylitol gum, her population of bugs changes from bad to good, which means she can't give the bad bugs to her child once he or she is born and the child has less cavities. Therefore, the better an expectant mother takes care of herself the better her child's teeth and gums will be.[38]

The list of snack foods and dietary products containing xylitol is rapidly expanding. The overwhelming majority of studies showed the protective effect of xylitol on tooth decay. In the face of the continuing high rate of caries in some populations in the presence of current dental caries prevention modalities, xylitol offers a potent tool that can have a significant impact.

Warning: As good as xylitol is for you, I need to remind you of two things: A common consensus seems to be a recommended dose of six to ten grams of xylitol, or three to five servings per day. Consuming too much xylitol can cause gastrointestinal problems. Some studies have shown that consuming more than 45 grams per day for children and more than 100 grams for adults per day can cause diarrhea.[39]

Even in small amounts, xylitol can be deadly to dogs. It doesn't take a whole lot of xylitol and the effects are rapid. If a dog digests any products containing xylitol, their owners should take them immediately to the veterinarian.[40]

5. Baking Soda

One of the most important parts of wellness is keeping your body in balance, and chief among these things is the pH. As you will see later, when we have a balanced pH of about seven the body is in balance.

Baking soda has been around for many years. It is a simple, cheap, and effective way to neutralize the acids of the mouth. Brushing with straight baking soda neutralizes the acids that bacteria need to break down your teeth and survive. If you want to increase the disease-fighting power of the baking soda you may also add a drop of essential oil or a teaspoon of salt for an effective tool to kill bacteria in the mouth.

This formula not only neutralizes the acids in the mouth and around the teeth but the salt is an effective way to kill the bad bugs. There are many toothpastes and powders that use baking soda as a carrier ingredient. It is a safe, effective, and gentle cleaner of stains on the teeth, and it neutralizes acids and helps fight gum disease and cavities.[41]

6. Arginine

If you want less cavities, researchers have found that people that eat arginine-rich foods and snacks get less cavities. Arginine is found in spinach, soy, seafood, nuts, seeds, dark chocolate, and seaweed. These make great snacks and meals for you and your family.[42]

CARIES MANAGEMENT PROTOCOL

Here is a real-life example to help you control, reverse, and prevent cavities and gum disease. Remember Jack, who lost a night's sleep fearing his dentist visit? How would you help him stop his cavities, reverse the cavities he may have, and prevent new cavities, allowing him to regain optimal health and vitality?

As Jack's parent, you would start with the most powerful tool you have: candy.

You would use the Loloz lollipop protocol of 20 lollipops 4 times a year. Every 3 months, you would have Jack get a professional cleaning and use an effective toothpaste immediately after every meal or snack, not just in the morning and evening.

You would add Dentiva or xylitol gum or candy to his lunch box, have xylitol products in the house, arginine-rich snack foods, and would avoid foods that alter his pH or Ca/P04 ratio.

You would reduce or eliminate all refined sugar, flour, or processed foods from the house and his diet. You would add raw fruits and vegetables, protein, and good fat sources, raw dairy, and fermented foods.

Here's what I would do, as a holistic dentist, to help take care of your son or daughter. It's called a Caries Management Protocol, which can be for anyone but it is specifically meant for cavity-prone or high-risk patients. It is a six-step process to stop cavities and reset the mouth to a healthier population of good bugs.

1. We begin with a professional cleaning by a hygienist who will use pumice polish to remove almost all the plaque in and around the teeth and gums, leaving a clean enamel surface, free of plaque, stain, bugs, and biofilm.
2. A two-minute iodine rinse with 10 percent Providine iodine. I use a peppermint or tutti fruity flavored iodine to help with the taste. This sterilizes all the plaque bugs and biofilm. It is much like rebooting a computer. We clear out all the bugs to reset the population and selectively let the good bugs back into the mouth. This is why I only use this as a last resort. It kills all the good bacteria in the mouth and only when the teeth are spotless because iodine stains the teeth.
3. Immediately after the professional cleaning the hygienist applies liberal amounts of MI paste to the teeth. The MI paste left on for three to five minutes helps strengthen the tooth enamel and starts to heal and repair any damaged enamel.
4. After the cleaning appointment, the child is instructed in how to use the Loloz lollipops and Dentiva lozenges.
5. I recommend applying MI paste to the teeth for two weeks—five minutes, three times a day with the last application at bedtime. This continues to strengthen the teeth, helps alkalinize the mouth, and protects the teeth at nighttime.
6. Oral hygiene at home includes an effective brushing technique with healthy toothpaste immediately after every meal or snack, irrigating

with effective solutions at least once a day, xylitol gum, candy, or mints (6 to 10 grams a day), and no in-between meal snacks, except raw nuts, seeds, fruits, or vegetables.[43]

ADJUNCTIVE THERAPIES

Besides these steps, there are many adjunctive therapies a person can use to avoid cavities and gum disease. Some of the most effective ones include a colloidal silver protocol two to four times a year, straight baking soda and/or a pinch of salt massage with a toothbrush in and around the teeth just before bedtime, hard cheese and raw nut snacks, high arginine foods (nuts, seeds, turkey, spinach, fish), increase the alkaline foods you eat, xylitol toothpastes, oral rinses, and mints, diluted bleach mouth rinse, sugar-free gums and candies, and a professional cleaning at least every three months for high cavity and gum disease risk patients.

REBUILDING THE TEETH NATURALLY

A healthy tooth is alive and vibrant. It may look like it just sits there quietly and solid, but the truth is it isn't. There is a constant outward flow of fluid and nutrients always flowing in the tooth. As we saw earlier, the hypothalamus starts one of these active processes. It stimulates the body's amazing process of rebuilding your teeth by sending down a message to your saliva glands.

The saliva is the storage house of all the building blocks of the teeth. The building blocks are caught up in the plaque layer surrounding your teeth and used to re-mineralize the tooth's structure.

The plaque on your teeth is good. It's an important part in the re-mineralizing of your teeth. It picks up the building blocks in your saliva and holds them close to the surface of your teeth.

If your pH level is above 4.5 and especially around seven or eight, then the construction and re-mineralizing of your teeth begins. Calcium and phosphorus combine to make hydroxyapatite crystals, which rebuild your teeth, reverse the cavity's damage, and strengthen your teeth from future attacks.[44]

Most of this rebuilding happens between meals, when the pH rises above 4.5 and the sugars and acids are gone and cleared off your teeth. Between meals the teeth and saliva rebuild your teeth, repair damage, and build strong teeth.

Let's follow the life of the tooth after a thorough professional cleaning to see how this plays out. Your teeth are spotless. All the plaque has been removed. The bug colonies have been broken up and washed away. The teeth are clean but bare and exposed.

Within 20 minutes, a thin layer of protein and carbohydrates coats the teeth. The teeth need this layer to help stay strong and rebuild. This layer is called "pellicle" or as the Bible calls it, "the skin of the teeth."[45]

This is the active rebuilding zone outside your teeth. Bathed in a pool of saliva with calcium and phosphorus, the immune system cells, oxygen, etc. the teeth use this protective and rebuilding layer to survive and thrive.

After your cleaning, some dentists like to make your teeth stronger by giving your teeth a fluoride treatment. They have found that the fluoride molecule can act in place of the calcium in your teeth to make them more resistant to an acid attack. Teeth with the fluoride molecule incorporated into the structure are more resistant to the acid attack then untreated natural enamel. The fluoride makes the surface of the teeth harder and stiffer than normal, but also more brittle.[46]

If you are using fluoride toothpaste, mouth rinse, or treatments, the fluoride is used as one of the building blocks to rebuild and repair your tooth. The fluorapatite crystal tooth structure is more solid, harder, and resistant to damage from the bad bacteria and their acid attack.

This would be a good thing for your teeth *if* the effects of the fluoride stopped here. But fluoride has a variety of bad effects in many parts of your body, not just your teeth. We will discuss the medical and biological damage this little fluorine molecule does in the human body. Here is a brief summary of the problems and some alternatives.

DENTISTRY'S BEST KEPT SECRET

For decades, dentists all over the world have claimed that fluoride is a safe, effective way of fighting cavities, but this is not true. *Fluoride is toxic. It has never been proven safe and is not as effective as you have been led to believe.*

Because it is one of the most electronegative elements on earth, fluoride is extremely reactive and is more toxic than lead and slightly less toxic than arsenic.

The National Federation of Federal Employees (local 2050 of the EPA) in Washington, D.C. states: "Our union member's review of the literature over the past 11 years has lead us to conclude that a causal link exists between fluoride and cancer, increased hip fractures, and damage to the central nervous system."[47]

In fact, fluoride has been linked to increases in fluorosis of the teeth and bones, cancers, genetic damage, bone pathology, brain, artery, and kidney damage, and lower IQs in children.

The U.S. Centers for Disease Control and the British Ministry of Health admit that no laboratory experiment has ever shown that fluoride in the drinking water is effective in reducing tooth decay. They also admit that there are no double blind epidemiological studies on humans showing that fluoridation reduces tooth decay. Three recent large-scale studies show no difference in decay rates of permanent teeth in fluoridated and non-fluoridated areas.[48]

You can rebuild your teeth with a product that rebuilds them like fluoride and makes them stronger *without* the damage to the rest of your body that fluoride causes.

An interesting product has hit the dental oral healthcare market and others may follow. Theodent is a toothpaste made from cacao extract, which harnesses the power of rennou, a revolutionary new additive to toothpaste that occurs naturally in the cacao plant, the source of chocolate.

Rennou works by growing the individual unit crystals in your enamel. These new crystals are four times larger and stronger than those found in normal enamel. Studies have shown that the ingredient in this apatite-forming toothpaste can enhance the re-mineralization of your teeth and may be a viable alternative to fluoride additives in commercial toothpastes. The theobromine ingredient has a re-mineralizing effect on enamel comparable to that of fluoride at even very small dosage levels.[49]

Theodent toothpaste is a more natural way to rebuild teeth as long as you avoid the fluoride version of the toothpaste. Non-fluoridated, Theodent Classic is a great alternative to fluoride. It is safe if swallowed, non-toxic, kid friendly, and the kid's version tastes like chocolate!

There are quite a few new toothpastes coming out in the market that claim to rebuild your teeth. Many of them use ingredients like strontium-chloride or potassium-nitrate. Sensodyne is a good example of these and can be very effective. These products use molecules that incorporate into the holes of your tooth's dentin tubules and make them stronger and less sensitive.

The problem with most of these products is that they like to add fluoride. They know that fluoride helps rebuild the teeth and their products market better if they contain it. The original Sensodyne in the pink box from Sweden did not contain fluoride. It was a safer product and could be recommended for sensitive teeth but not now, as it contains the fluoride, as do most other products.

Look for new products coming out while avoiding products with fluoride that don't control the pH of your mouth. In between meals should be a time of rest and rebuilding between acid attacks. Keep your body in balance and the body knows how to repair, rebuild, and stay strong itself.

REBUILDING YOUR GUMS NATURALLY

If you have had or have gum disease you have seen the level of your gums recede. The destruction of tissue and bone during the gum disease process is significant and usually happens pain-free over the years. Bad bugs and the body's immune system are at war and the products they use to fight each other and the exchange of dangerous chemicals they release during the fight silently destroy the gum tissue and bone around your teeth.

Even if the bad bugs are eradicated, the gums can look like they've been pulled down, exposing the roots of your teeth. We have no way to grow the gums back up the tooth, but we have many ways to heal the tissue and strengthen the remaining bone.

Periodontists (gum specialists) have gotten very good at pulling existing gum tissue back up to the tooth with microsurgery (bone and tissue graphs). They have many ways to fill in bone holes and pockets and have achieved miraculous results.

They can use bone from cows, cadavers, and artificial bone, and/or the most natural option—your own bone. This is taken from your jaw, tori (bumps of extra bone some people have), or a bone from other parts of the body. If harvested from your own bone, your body can do amazing things to give you back the bone level you used to have.

One of the most exciting new procedures is low-level laser treatment, which uses very low levels of lasers at 1 to 2 watts of power. This is one of the safest therapies we have available for killing bad bugs, repairing tissue, and healing the body.[50]

WHAT CAN YOU DO NOW?

Once you have had a good professional cleaning and verified through the use of a phase contrast microscope that you no longer have bad bugs, what is the next step to healing and rebuilding your gums and bone?

To sum up our lessons in this chapter, use effective toothpaste, irrigate with an effective solution in your irrigator, see your dentist/hygienist regularly, eat a healthy diet, and use supplements for nutrients not found in your foods.

Enjoy the Loloz lollipops twice a year, use Dentiva when you can't brush, and add MI paste for sensitivity or as needed to repair your own teeth.

Although there are many helpful tools available now to help you keep and maintain your teeth and gums, these are the bare essentials. See the appendix for a list of things to use and where to look to find a dentist by you that can help you achieve optimal health and vitality.

In the future, there should be less need for dentists, less drilling and needles, and less pain. We should be able to treat patients with minimally invasive dentistry with minimal cavities and gum disease. Using a combination of herbs, essential oils, and the foods found in our marvelous world, we can treat gum disease and cavities before they start, prevent disease, and live a life of optimal health and vitality—with beautiful smiles.

2

From Our Mind to Our Mouth: Holistic Dentistry and the Medical Health Connection

This is our first step in a grand adventure. We have packed our suitcases in the car with the essentials we need, driven to our destination, and are about to get out of the car and explore the interconnection between our teeth and gums and the rest of our body, how one affects the other in multiple directions. This is information—some old, some new—that I don't have time to tell my patients during their first brief dental exam. I am excited to share it with you here, as I feel confident that these ideas and concepts can make a positive difference in your life, by expanding your view of the body, how it affects your dental health, and vice versa.

We will investigate the immune system, how your mouth is affected by chronic inflammation in your body, the dangers of oxidative stress and toxins, and how cavities and gum disease are host meditated bacterial infections, which means that *you*, who are hosting these invaders, are more important and need careful, special attention.

I will show you the biggest problems that your teeth cause in the rest of the body. For example, mercury fillings cause six health problems and root canals negatively affect the rest of your body because they block meridians and release toxins in to your blood.

We also show how gum disease and cavities can cause heart disease, diabetes, obesity, arthritis, respiratory infections, cancer, and an assortment of other chronic illnesses. We share information about the poisons the Federal Drug Administration (FDA) allows in your toothpaste, the association between dental implants and cancer, how many chronic illnesses are caused by three conditions you can control, and why the anesthetics used every day by traditional dentists may be one of the most poisonous products in dentistry.

Before we go into detail on any of these topics, I want to provide you with a brief history of dental healthcare and give you an idea of where we are headed in this adventure.

FROM BARBERS TO BACTERIA:
A BRIEF HISTORY OF DENTAL HEALTHCARE

The earliest modern dentists were local barbers, who kept a small arsenal of herbal remedies and pastes. Since they did not know what caused bad teeth, and often suspected worms, their solution was frequently extraction. This practice was based on a surgical model of disease and treatment. These "dentists" eventually tried to fill lost teeth and holes using carpentry methods with various materials, such as wood, ivory, and gold. As new materials and chemicals came on to the scene, dentists started to be more professional and formed a professional organization in an effort to obtain credibility and stature. But as they continued following in the footsteps of the medical establishment, which influenced many of their ideas about disease and treatment techniques, this solidified the medical model of dental healthcare.

We've moved beyond the surgical model, but unfortunately, the medical model is still the norm, including physical manipulation, rebuilding structures, and finding new drugs and chemicals to treat symptoms of dental disease. All of these are still quite common, such as the use of commercial toothpastes, flossing, fluoride, mercury fillings, root canals, bridges, and complete dentures. For many dentists, their adventure has stopped here, perhaps because they fear new ideas, looking different, or challenging old concepts, opting instead to remain content with the status quo, with little desire to venture into uncharted territory. This approach has kept some dentists and

Table 2.1. History of Dental Healthcare

Surgical Model (1880s)	Medical Model (1930s)	Holistic Dental Model (1960s)	Spirit/Energy Model (1990s)
Worms	Non-specific plaque	Specific plaque	Whole body/ environ
Herbal remedies	Bacteria & plaque	Bad bugs, biofilm	Energy/balance
Pastes	Toothpaste/floss	Diet, pH, Ca/PO4 ratio	Love/fear
Extractions	PXS, fillings	Toxins, meridians	Christ conscience
Some replacements	Drugs/chemicals	Minimally invasive	Tx temple, others, God

their patients stuck in the medical model of dental healthcare, which focuses on the signs and symptoms of disease and rarely address the root causes, let alone connect the emotional and spiritual influences on our physical wellness.

On our adventure, we step into the *holistic dental model* of healthcare. By looking at the whole host—the entire person—we can expand our view of the body beyond the mouth.

Newer, more open-minded practitioners look at the physical body of the patient and the world around that individual for the primary cause of poor health and disease. That includes diet, pH, CaPO4 ratios, fluid flow inside the tooth, meridians, and energy flows in the body. This is the key to determining the primary causes of disease and imbalances.

As we proceed on our adventure, we will also encounter the *spiritual/energy model* of creating and maintaining vitality and good health.

I will show how the medical connection works, with examples from biology, chemistry, biochemistry, and physics. These connections are simpler than you may think and you will learn easy tools to help heal and maintain balance.

BIOLOGY

We presented the anatomy of the teeth in the previous chapter, including the gums and bone that surround the teeth. Now, let's expand on the anatomy and our understanding of how the teeth and the rest of the body interact.

Inside the teeth is living pulp, which consists of arteries, veins, and nerves. Blood from the rest of your body flows into each tooth and circulates again throughout your body. That means all the blood, oxygen, nutrients, and immune system cells in your body's blood are constantly affecting your teeth, gums, and bones.

For example, calcium and phosphorus minerals constantly enter your tooth pulp to rebuild your teeth. A lack of the proper nutrients, oxygen, or changes in the pH of your blood, can negatively affect the teeth and gums.

If you are not eating the right foods, getting enough oxygen, or are generally out of balance, your teeth cannot repair themselves and you will become vulnerable to cavities and gum disease. This concept is especially important for the gums. They are pink because they are richly supplied with blood vessels. Any change in your blood's pH, nutrients, or oxygen levels will affect the gums and how they fight off possible unwelcome invaders.

Cavities and gum disease are host-mediated bacterial infections.

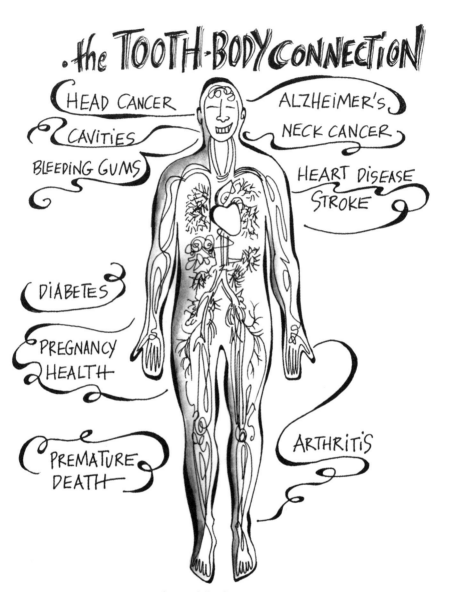

The tooth/body connection

THE DISCOVERY OF VITAMIN C

Scurvy is a particularly stereotypical disease, characterized by apathy, weakness, easy bruising, skin hemorrhages, friable bleeding gums, and swollen legs. Untreated patients may die. Scurvy is due to a deficiency of an essential food factor—ascorbic acid, or vitamin C, which when taken in adequate quantities, completely prevents and cures the disease, so that now it is rare. Long intercontinental voyages at sea began in the late sixteenth century and sailors eventually discovered that scurvy could be cured and prevented by oranges and lemons. However, most physicians ignored this lay therapy in favor of ancient theories and useless polypharmacy. Public recognition of the value of citrus fruits came from thoughtful eighteenth century ships' surgeons, especially James Lind, whose 1753 Treatise of the Scurvy inspired his successors to persuade the British admiralty in the 1790s to abolish naval scurvy with the juice of European lemons.

Albert Szent-Gyorgyi, from 1928 to 1933, was the first to isolate the anti-scurvy factor, hexuronic acid, derived from the adrenal cortex. Since the term scorbutic pertains to scurvy, it was first named ascorbic acid, until it became designated later as vitamin C.[1]

VITAMIN C AND YOU

Low levels of vitamin C in the blood will negatively affect your gums and you will see more bleeding. Vitamin C is used to build the cell walls of the blood vessels with collagen. Without an adequate amount of this vitamin, the collagen parts of the blood vessel walls become weak and leak, and can be traced back to imbalances in the rest of the body.

If you have gum disease, the body tries to fight it off by flooding the area with immune system fighters, white blood cells, and inflammation cells. They get there through the blood and you can see this as the gum tissue becomes swollen and red.

Remember: teeth are alive. They don't just sit there and chew food. There is a constant flow of nutrients, oxygen, and cells coming and going from the teeth to the rest of the body. For example, if your tooth is infected, this infection goes to all the rest of the body through these same blood vessels.

Besides the teeth and gums, all your teeth are held in place by bone. Bone is not just sitting there, either. Your bone is an active factory, constantly making new blood, red blood cells, and immune system cells. Your bone needs nutrients and healthy immune system cells from the rest of the body to fight infection, repair and rebuild itself, fight off cancer, balance your pH and Ca/PO4 ratio, along with many other functions.

If your body is low in calcium, magnesium, or Vitamin D, your bones will not have the building blocks they need to repair and rebuild. If there is constant, chronic inflammation and infection around a bone, it will lose the fight. Over time, it will dissolve and fall away from your teeth. Receding gums and bones are the result of this, and that results in gum disease.

Your teeth, gums, and bones are intimately connected to the rest of your body!

Consider what happens with a cavity. An infected tooth can be extremely painful and even life threatening. Infected teeth flood the body through the blood stream with bacteria, poisons, and chronic inflammation that can affect any tissue downstream. These products flow out of the teeth into the veins, through the heart, and to every part of the body. The amount of pus released from an abscessed tooth can be up to two tablespoons, and this is poured into your bloodstream every day if you have an infection. The pus, filled with bacteria and white blood cells, permeates the rest of the body and can make you get very sick. Malaise, fever, and fatigue begin to take over the body—besides the pain. Some of these bugs can grow on your heart and shut off the flow of blood to your body. Some can get into your head's circulatory system and cause Alzheimer's and even fatal brain infections.

New research is showing how the gums, teeth, and bones can affect the rest of the body. Gingivitis sounds mild and easy to take care of, but if it is not fought off correctly it progresses into periodontitis, or gum disease, which can affect the rest of the body. Researchers have found the gums to be part of the cause for heart disease, diabetes, obesity, arthritis, respiratory infections, pancreatic and liver cancer, and many other chronic illnesses.[2]

The bugs that harbor in infected gum pockets have an open channel into your blood stream, and they easily double their numbers every 5 hours. You can have trillions of bugs in these gums and they have to go someplace. We swallow them or share them with others, but most of them travel into our blood stream. This infection sets up chronic inflammation, which spreads all over the body. The body tries to fight these bugs, and in the process destroys nearby tissue and organs. Infected gums are devastating to the balance of your whole body. That is why it is so important to take care of them. You need to break up the colonies of bad bugs and get rid of them.[3]

A holistic dentist can help you stay healthy.

He or she can check for bad bugs with a microscope, offer thorough, non-surgical cleanings, and healthy effective products, while also teaching you how to take care of yourself and provide follow-up to see if you are doing a good job.

ENDODONTIC
ROOT CANAL TREATMENT

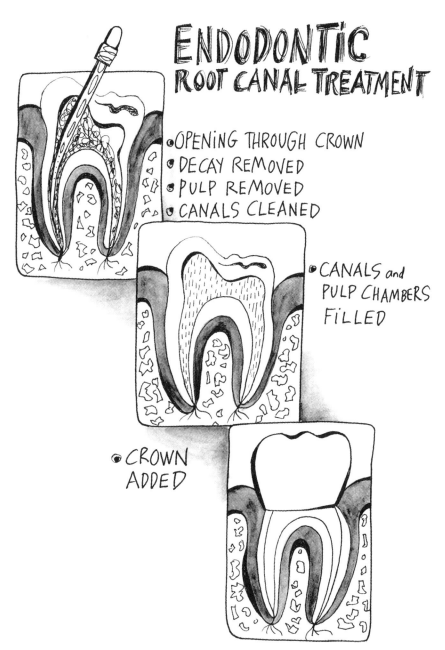

- OPENING THROUGH CROWN
- DECAY REMOVED
- PULP REMOVED
- CANALS CLEANED

- CANALS and PULP CHAMBERS FILLED

- CROWN ADDED

Root canal treated tooth

We've made it this far without bringing up the dreaded issue of root canals, which unfortunately have become the bane of too many people's existence. It's not a laughing matter, at all, I'm sad to say, because a root canal treated tooth can affect your health in negative ways.

Consider the fact that dentistry is one of the few healing professions that routinely leave a dead body part inside the body. Most doctors and health-care practitioners remove dead tissue from the body whenever possible. Dentists do not.

When you get a root canal, the inside of the tooth is opened up and hallowed out. This process is meant to take care of the infection trapped inside the tooth and stop it from spreading in the body. While a normal type of root canal tries to sterilize the inside of the tooth and its large pulp chamber with bleach, lasers, and ozone, they have a hard time sterilizing the smaller roots, or "legs" of the tooth. Here there are thousands of tiny tubules going down the roots of the tooth that are filled with millions of bacteria. Lined up end to end, these tubules would end up approximately 3 miles long—all filled with bacteria during a root canal.

These bacteria, which are missed by conventional root canal treatments, change their metabolism when trapped inside the tooth. They mutate into anaerobic bacteria and release poisons into the tooth's thousands of tubules, which in turn release their poisons out of the tooth roots into the surrounding bone and bloodstream.

In his book, *Healing Is Voltage,* Jerry Tennant, MD, MD(H) describes the link between cancer, disease, and chronic infections, by looking at what affect the oxygen, enzyme systems, and voltage of the body's cells. He believes that none of the environmental factors most doctors worry about are as destructive as a tooth, which has been through a root canal. He believes that teeth are at one end of our acupuncture meridians, and when they are dead and infected from a root canal it is like pulling the plug on that whole electrical system. Dr. Tennant thinks that nothing can be done to ever overcome the toxins from a root canal, that it must be removed and the infected bone cleared.[4]

In a lecture given at the International Society for Orthomolecular Medicine in Vancouver, Canada, Thomas Levy, MD, JD gave a lecture on "Oral Pathogens as a Common Cause of Chronic Disease." He feels that *all* infection and toxins—without exception—cause cell tissue damage and produce symptoms by increasing oxidative stress.

Dental infections and dental toxicity are involved in oxidative stress. When pathogens in the mouth are allowed to magnify, substantial chronic disease can ensue, led prominently by heart disease, cancer, and autoimmune system diseases. Primary sources of oral infection and toxicity are root canaled teeth, abscessed teeth, chronic periodontal infection/inflammation, cavitations, gangrene from old extraction sites, chronically infected tonsils, infected dental implants, and toxic metals.

In a study examining 5,000 extracted root canal-treated teeth, 100 percent of them had bad bugs and highly potent pathogen-related toxins. All root canal-treated teeth continually produce endogenous toxins as the bugs grow. Root canals that have been "identified" as infected have been found to have fungi, viruses, and over 450 different types of bacteria in them.[5]

More and more research is being done on the effect of the root canals and their poisons leaking into the rest of the body.

Years ago, a concerned dentist tried to improve on the disinfection of these teeth in an effort to kill all the bugs hiding in the tubules. He found a cement that expanded into the tubules, which could affect almost all the bugs in the tooth.

Endocal (formally Biocalex) is a sealer cement, which can be used to more thoroughly sterilize teeth. It has been tested and used for over 30 years. Therefore, if you need a root canal or really want to save a dead tooth, go to a specialist and have an Endocal type root canal. After it is finished, I recommend you follow-up with an evaluation and treatment by an acupuncturist. This is needed to open up and rebalance the acupuncture meridians of the body. That's because the infection and the root canal treatment affect the body's energy channels or acupuncture meridians by blocking the energy flowing through these meridians. Chinese medicine and acupuncture have treated the body differently than Western medicine for thousands of years. Based on a system of treating these energy channels and the flow of the body, they have treated diseases successfully for a long time and continue to do so.

The teeth are at the top of these meridians, which flow up the back of the body, through the head and back down the front of the body. Each of your teeth is connected to one of these energy channels, so when they are infected or root canaled they block the energy flowing through this meridian.

Dentist and acupuncturist working together have come up with charts that show these connections and which tooth affects which meridian and organ system.

Metal teeth implants may cause the same blockages and imbalances that infected root canaled teeth suffer. There is no research on the body's reaction to implants or the conditions that may be caused by the placement of an artificial metal screw in your jawbone.

We have seen cases of cancer forming after implant surgeries. Two recent articles in dental journals have questioned the link between metal implants and oral cancer. Back in 2008, the first dental case of malignant cancer associated with a dental implant was reported in *The Journal of the American Dental Association*'s August 2008 issue. A maxillary osteosarcoma developed in a

DENTAL MERIDIANS
YOUR TEETH and BODY CONNECTIONS

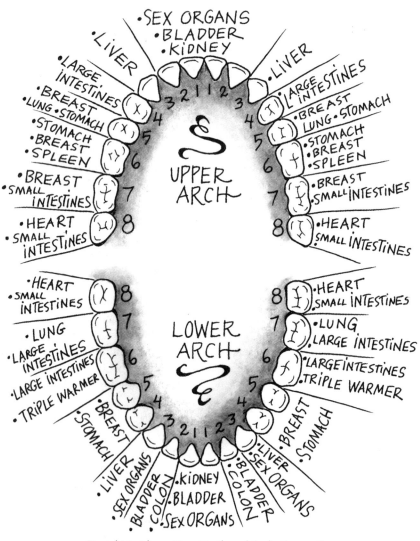

Dental Meridians: Your Teeth and Body Connection

38-year-old woman after receiving a titanium dental implant. They treated the cancer by cutting off her jaw and giving her systemic chemotherapy.[6]

In 2011, other lesions, multifocal oral melanoacanthoma, and melanotic maculas developed in a 63-year-old woman after implant surgery. The surgery could have been causal or incidental to the appearance of these lesions. Dentists and patients need to be aware of these rare but devastating complications due to dental implants and ask for possible options.[7]

The field of dental implants is young and there is very little research on their health consequences to know if they are safe. I would consider the placement of dental implants in the jawbone as a still unproven technique and an experimental dental health care practice. I may be old-fashioned in this regard, but I still prefer dental bridges made with solid porcelain or zirconia. I consider them a better option for replacement of most teeth spaces.

CHEMISTRY

The next connection between your teeth, gums, and the rest of the body falls in the realm of chemistry. How do all the fillings, crowns, bridges, and root canals in your mouth affect the rest of the body? How do the ingredients in your toothpaste and mouthwash affect your body?

Many books tell you about the poisons in mercury fillings, root canaled teeth, or nickel and beryllium in your crowns. While this information is important, and I will provide a short summary of these affects to show you the connections, I do not think it is vital to dwell on them. The focus on physical materials and their influence is not as important as the fear these concerns cause and the importance of the emotional and spiritual influences on the rest of the body.

For example, I knew one healthcare practitioner whose wife became chronically ill. She had a mouth full of mercury fillings but because of a lack of finances and advanced age they were not able to replace all of them. Instead, he was able to heal her with an emotional and spiritual method *without* changing any of her fillings and dental work.

Here was a spiritual healing practitioner using prayer, intention, and God's power and love to help heal his wife. He treated her with these techniques and never replaced her dentistry. Her body regained its balance through emotional and spiritual healing.

Subsequent tests for mercury and other metals showed that she was clear. It was as if the mercury and metals were gone and did not negatively affect her body any longer. Her husband facilitated, or was a conduit, for God's power and love, which reversed the affects and influences of a chemical like mercury and brought her body back into balance and good health.

This demonstrates how an emphasis on fearing our physical environment is misguided. If someone is positively focused on loving their body and others around them, they will achieve balance and health.

DENTAL FILLINGS AND CROWNS

If you have silver-mercury fillings in your teeth, keep in mind that they are releasing mercury vapor into your body all day and every day and surface area rust particles of mercury are being worn off and swallowed at a regular rate. The mercury vapor is breathed into your lungs and respiratory tract and absorbed into all the tissues it contacts. The mercury crosses over to your bloodstream in the lungs and travels throughout your body.[8]

Mercury seeks sulfur to bind itself to and finds this in the sulfur-rich proteins in the tissues of your body, largely found in your kidneys, liver, brain, and nervous system. This mercury interferes with your body's function, destroys tissue, kills cells, and has been proven to have many of the following affects:

Depression: By inhibiting dopamine, noradrenaline, and serotonin, causing hopelessness, lack of focus, concentration, and apathy.
Fatigue: By interfering with enzymes and binding with hemoglobin, it reduces oxygen transport in the body.
Allergies: By interfering with digestive enzymes and zinc absorption.
Headaches: By antibiotic effects in the GI tract, leading to fungus, fermenting foods, and toxin release. Anoxia lowers oxygen in the blood and by allergy tightening on the meningeal system.
Memory loss: By binding with metallothionein and competing with Mg and Mn. Mercury also causes the formation of neurofibrillary tangles and amyloid plaque in the brain, which are two diagnostic markers for Alzheimer's disease.
Candida: By antibiotic affect in the GI tract, candida becomes overgrown.[9]

Scientific studies have identified dental mercury as a potential cause or exacerbating factor in many other conditions as well, including Amyotrophic lateral sclerosis, antibiotic resistance, autism spectrum disorders, autoimmune disorders, cardiovascular problems, hearing loss, kidney disease, multiple sclerosis, oral lichen planus, Parkinson's disease, reproductive dysfunction, suicidal ideations, and thyroiditis.[10]

METALS IN DENTISTRY

Beryllium: This is used in partial dentures and cheap crowns. Signs and symptoms include incurable lung disease (Berylliosis), caused by inhaling dust or through skin contact, which reduces ATP intra-cellular activity and lowers cellular energy metabolism, causing a formation of granulomas, usually in the lungs, skin, lymph, or liver.

Nickel: This is used in cheap crowns and bridges, posts, pins, and some temporary crowns. Signs and symptoms include cancer (especially lung), caused by damaging the body's RNA, which is needed for cell replication. Nickel also causes allergies in 33 percent of women and 12 percent of men who have been exposed to it, as well as immune system problems, such as lupus, arthritis, ulcers, endometriosis, and digestive system inflammation.

Aluminum: This is used in cheap permanent and temporary crowns. Signs and symptoms include Alzheimer's, senile dementia, seizures, caused by destroying vitamins, lowering phosphate levels, causing weakness in the bones, teeth, and muscles, and it also affects cytochrome P450 and metallothionein detox systems.[11]

ROOT CANAL TREATED TEETH

In addition to your dental fillings and crowns, your root canal treated teeth also affect the rest of the body by releasing toxic chemicals and destroying enzyme systems throughout the body. Some of the proteins present in the fluid around the teeth, which indicate inflammation, include alkaline phosphate (human and bacterial), human antibodies, human serum albumin, human serum transferring, and many unidentified proteins. They are normally present in only trace amounts in samples taken from healthy tissue. These proteins, in contrast to bacterial toxins, remain largely confined to the sites of production. Their presence indicates infection.[12]

Protein *enzymes* are toxins that can spread from the sites of production to other sites in the mouth and the rest of the body. These chemicals can cause imbalance and disease conditions far away from where a tooth underwent a root canal.

If you have any chronic health problems, especially a cancer history or other assault on the body from chemicals, then the added assault of toxins leaking out of your root-canaled teeth may be too much for your body to handle. There are many alternative doctors you can ask about the possible health consequences of a root canal in your specific case and if you would be better off having the tooth extracted.

ANESTHETICS IN DENTISTRY

The anesthetics used in dentistry are another powerful chemical introduced to your body. Are they safe? Most of the anesthetics in dentistry are made from coal tar and its derivatives. Dentists inject a large dose of these chemicals into your body during procedures. These anesthetics are an amazing development in dentistry, allowing complex surgical procedures in a painless manner.

But the chemicals injected into your body have physical consequences.
Let's consider some of the chemicals being used today:

Lidocaine: A health risk for patients with hepatic (liver) disease because of their inability to metabolize it normally. Patients allergic to para-aminobenzoic acid (procaine, tetracaine, benzocaine, etc.) have shown a cross sensitivity to lidocaine. A minor metabolite in lidocaine, 2, 6-xylidine, has been found to be carcinogenic in rats. Other systemic reactions may include light- headedness, nervousness, apprehension, euphoria, confusion, dizziness, drowsiness, tinnitus, blurred vision, vomiting, sensations of heat, cold, and numbness, twitching, tremors, convulsions, unconsciousness, and respiratory depression and arrest.[13]

Septocaine: Years ago in Germany, a company was looking for an alternative anesthetic and developed an anesthetic that was not derived from coal tar. Septocaine was chemically made, and did not contain the cancer-causing ingredients that can be found in other anesthetics. It can be a great choice for many dental procedures—instead of Lidocaine. It has not been shown to be associated with higher risks of cancer. I suggest you look for a dentist familiar with Septocaine, who provides it as an option for dental treatments that require anesthetics.

On a positive note, you might look for a dentist that prays over the products in his or her practice and blesses the dental materials he or she uses. A blessing and positive intention can physically change the products to have only positive effects on the body.

By this point, you may be wandering what I have used for my dental work, if all these products are so detrimental to your health. We are blessed to be born in to a time of healthy alternatives for all these unhealthy, chemical-laden products. There are hundreds of safe products available to all dentists and they can be used instead of the prior unhealthy products.

So how do you choose which product to use?
Which product would be best for your mouth and body?

There are a few ways. Some dentists and healthcare providers do testing on dental products by looking at the way your body reacts to various products or ingredients. The testing machines can look at your body's immune system cells response, weakness in muscles, frequency or energy response, and many other functional test responses. Much of the testing can give accurate results, but they are very dependent on the practitioner and limited to the number of products tested. Many of the practitioners may not be as accurate as others, but how would you know?

Even if you have an accurate practitioner doing energy, frequency, or muscle testing, there are hundreds of thousands different products in dentistry to test for, and the number is growing. Even if you pick the right product, these results can change over time with different results.

I prefer to use an immunological blood reactivity test, which is based more on your body's reaction to various ingredients, instead of a practitioner's observation of subjective results. This test uses 22,000 commonly used products in dentistry and measures your body's response to them. I consider it the best, most affordable, and reliable testing of dental products on the market today.

This Clifford Reactivity Test observes your body's physical reaction to 94 chemical groups and families of compounds and looks at passive antibody detection by the precipitin method—present at or above a relevant threshold to eliminate noise effects from casual contacts. It is looking at your body's IgG and IgM response to these 94 chemical groups and compounds.[14]

The cost is minimal and easy to administer. The results are easy to use and reliably accurate. I have used this testing with more than 600 patients with sensitivity issues and find them to be reliable. There is no best way to test for the body's reaction to any product commonly used in dentistry today, but this test currently comes the closest.

With this testing, you can select safe options from the many resins, porcelains, golds, zirconias, and glues used in dentistry today. All of these products can leach out or affect the body. This is the best way to pick your options, especially if you have multiple sensitivities.

For example, one of the chemicals in these products, Bisphenol A, which can leach out of dental products, has caught the attention of the media. It can have negative effects by mimicking the structure of a female sex hormone in the body. The complex chemicals in resin, glues, and bonding agents can have this chemical or leach this reaction product into the body. Currently, all of the newest products in dentistry do not contain Bisphenol A and have significantly cut down on chemicals that can react to create this chemical.[15]

A WORD ON FLOURIDE

Many of our dental products contain another chemical that can have deleterious effects on the body and is not necessary in the products themselves.

This chemical is fluoride.

Dental manufacturers tend to add this chemical to almost all their products because dentists are more likely to buy the products when they do. It is now a little difficult to find good dental products that do not have added fluoride in them. Many dentists actively look for fluoride in their resins and glues. Most of these dentists are looking for products that actively release fluoride ions to try to stop future cavities in their patients.

We touched on the myths around fluoride before but let's consider what it does as part of your fillings, glues, and toothpastes as it enters the rest of your body.

Whether you are swallowing toothpaste after brushing your teeth, rinsing with a fluoride mouth rinse, or swallowing the fluoride leaching out of your dental work, fluoride gets taken up by your GI tract and enters your bloodstream. From there, it has access to your whole body. The small size and highly reactive nature of the fluoride ions helps it get everywhere and binds irreversibly to many places in the body.

The International Association of Oral and Medical Toxicology declares in one of its position papers that "the present U.S. E.P.A. maximum contaminant level for water (4ppm) and the recommendation for drinking water fluoridation (1ppm) will produce a measurable increased risk of cancer, hip fracture, dental fluorosis, and neurological impairment and virtually assures the development of stages I and II skeletal fluorosis in many individuals exposed to these levels of fluoride in their drinking water. The International Academy of Oral Medicine and Toxicology (IAOMT) PHG (Public Health Goal) for fluoride is appropriately zero."[16]

Let me repeat: fluoride is a no-no.

CHEMICALS IN DENTAL HYGIENE PRODUCTS

What chemicals are you swallowing and absorbing every day by using your preferred toothpaste and mouthwash? Do they have an effect on the rest of your body?

We know that fluoride comes in many forms, such as SnF_2, sodium fluoride, sodium monofluorophosphate, and others. Some have pyrophosphates, sodium lauryl sulfates, propylene glycol, sodium saccharin, and many others. These are all swallowed, absorbed by the body, and can affect many other tissues and organs.

Triclosan, a favorite ingredient in Colgate's toothpastes, became a banned pesticide by the FDA in 2016. If you use it, you are voluntarily putting a banned pesticide into your mouth, where the rest of your body will absorb it.[17] Triclosan may kill the bad bugs that cause gum disease, but it does not stop there. It kills both good and bad bugs and keeps on doing damage to the rest of your body. In fact, it has been shown in a number of scientific studies to disrupt the endocrine system, promote breast cancer cell proliferation, reduce fertility, lower sperm count and motility, and has been connected to bacterial resistance.[18]

There is a reason why so many toothpastes, especially those containing fluoride, carry a warning label on them, telling you that if you swallow the product, you should contact the poison control center immediately. Please take a closer look at these warning labels. In fact, it would probably be best to avoid using toothpaste that requires a warning label in the first place.

As I mentioned earlier, I would recommend natural effective ingredients, and ingredients that if swallowed and absorbed by the body would not cause health problems. I recommend essential oils, herbs, and other natural ingredients that kill the bad bugs and leave the good bugs alone.

BIOCHEMISTRY

Let's examine the effects your mouth has on the rest of the body and how your body also affects your mouth. Though related to simple inorganic chemistry, biochemistry is a little more complex and deals with an intricate relationship between the chemicals you are exposed to and your body's own functions. Most of these reactions involve how the body affects the mouth through changing conditions inside it.

The first is pH balance. We saw before that your teeth tend to dissolve and a cavity can start when the pH of the plaque on your teeth falls below pH = 4.5. We saw that many short-term exposures to snack foods can immediately drop the pH of the mouth to below 4.5.[19]

The body has a direct effect on controlling the long-term pH level of your mouth.[20] Though the science is complex, I want to provide you with a summary to help explain some of the greatest effects the body has on the mouth.

PARTNERING WITH YOUR DENTIST

We can offer a multitude of help to deal with the conditions and interactions inside the body and describe the wide variety of healthcare practitioners who are available.

The first is a holistic and alternative minded MD.

Holistic MDs can address concerns you have about your mouth that might have a medical consequence. MDs can diagnosis and treat medical conditions, such as diabetes, heart disease, and bacterial imbalances that affect your teeth and gums. They can treat oxidative stress and chronic inflammation (that we will get to in the next chapter) that is a direct cause of many chronic illnesses, including gum disease. They can pull toxins out of the body and detox your tissues with chelation therapy. They can prescribe nutritional supplements, give oxygen to your tissues, and supply your body with many of the nutrients it needs to achieve optimal health and vitality.

A medical doctor can answer specific questions about replacing fillings and root canals. A good partnership between you and both a holistic dentist and MD can form a powerful team.

Naturopaths and NMDs can be a great resource for a variety of health issues and concerns. Diet, supplements, nutritional support, and functional balance can all be best figured out through the diagnosis and testing that these professionals can perform for you.

Osteopathic physicians (DOs) provide a wealth of information on the body, diet, functional balance, and structural issues. The use of healthcare practitioners is sometimes needed to know what you don't know. We all know a lot of things but we don't know what we don't know. Sometimes, we need instruction and partnerships with others that may know more.

Acupuncturists have a different viewpoint of the body than Western medical doctors. They have been using their Eastern medicine type of healthcare for thousands of years. Acupuncture herbs, diet, harmony, and balance of energies are all helpful for a vast array of conditions that Western medicine cannot address. For example, acupuncture can address the far-reaching effects of a root canaled tooth, implant, or infection of a tooth on the rest of the body.

Chiropractors and dentists should always be working together. The balance of one's bite can greatly affect muscles and nerves in the body—all the way down to the feet. Subluxations of the spinal column, bones of the skeleton, and affected nerves can greatly affect the whole body. Cooperation between the two healthcare fields is necessary to achieve and maintain balance throughout the entire body.

Craniosacral chiropractors specifically work with the bones of the head and neck and their direct influences on the teeth and jaws of their clients. Bridges and partial dentures across the sutures of the head can affect the health and circulation of your head. The need for communication with the chiropractor and your dentist in TMJD problems is absolutely necessary and has recently been taught more and more than ever before.

Reiki and healing touch practitioners can sometimes diagnosis and treat conditions that have not been resolved with routine dentistry and medicine. The effective use of healing energy from the hands and manipulation of these practitioners can make a big difference in the body's response and healing imbalances. I have seen amazing healing from many of those gifted individuals.

THE PERILS OF CHRONIC INFLAMMATION AND OXIDATIVE STRESS

The physical root causes of most of our civilized diseases are chronic inflammation and oxidative stress. Heart disease, diabetes, obesity, Alzheimer's disease, dementia, gum disease, arthritis, and cancer, can be caused by these two physical conditions.

Chronic inflammation is the long-term stimulation of the body's immune system fighting off some condition. Think of it as a fire burning inside you that never goes out.[21]

Oxidative stress is the breakdown of the body's systems and can be thought of as your body rusting and falling apart.[22]

Both of these are conditions that affect the entire body.

For example, the chronic inflammation of your gums as part of having periodontal disease spreads through your bloodstream and into the tissues of every part of your body. The inflammatory cells and proteins mediators have far-reaching effects on the tissues, organs, and systems—all over your body.

Gum disease contributes to the breakdown of your blood vessels, heart, and organs, which in turn affect the gums. Gum disease is linked to obesity and pregnancy issues, and these conditions affect other systems cascading around the body, causing imbalance and disease.

WE ARE ONE

The teeth and gums affect the rest of the body and the rest of the body affects your teeth and gums. They are interconnected and we need both to be in balance for optimal health and vitality. The physical parts of your body are all connected through the blood vessels, nerves, lymphatic systems, and energy pathways.

A good example of the positive connection between your mouth and the rest of your body can be found through a typical dental cleaning. Every time you go for a good thorough cleaning, the hygienist is getting rid of bad bugs, breaking up biofilm, oxidizing the tissues, and removing toxins. After this treatment, your whole body feels the positive affects. You have lower levels of bad bugs in your blood stream, more oxygen, less oxidative stress, less chronic inflammation, and better balance.

In addition to all the other healthcare providers we mentioned before that can partner with you to obtain optimal health, *do not forget your dental hygienist*. He or she is getting you healthier every time you receive a thorough dental cleaning.

Aside from your dentist, hygienist, and other healthcare practitioners, remember that *you* are the biggest factor in achieving optimal health and vitality.

Our next chapter goes over one of the most important factors in obtaining optimal balance. You have ultimate control over it, and it can be the biggest, most important part of the physical body. That topic is nutrition and your diet.

3

Nutrition: How "Friendly" Foods Affect Your Teeth and Gums

A journey through this chapter will show how foods control your health and play a crucial role in forming or avoiding disease. For example, when the body experiences a real imbalance in nutrition it will also affect the teeth, and only then will you start developing a cavity.

We'll begin by explaining the essential nutrients everyone needs for optimal health and vitality and the exact effects of nutrition on one's general wellness—from diet, pH, and Ca/PO4 ratio to the dangers of sugar, processed foods, and oils. This also includes the importance of good, clean water, fats that heal and fats that kill, proteins important to build and maintain a strong immune system, and how simple and complex carbohydrates affect our bodies. We also explain the role of essential vitamins and minerals in creating healthy teeth and gums and how they can repair themselves through a regimen of wise choices. Finally, we explain the dangers of fad diets, the advantages of the Body Type diet, Zone diet concepts, and Dr. Ed Group's helpful diet suggestions and detox programs.

WHAT SHOULD I EAT?

Proper nutrition can enable your teeth and gums to thrive. Anyone can learn to eat the right foods and *never* have another cavity, gum disease, or crooked teeth. Knowing what you should eat will help you stay balanced and whole.

As your body grows and develops, it rebuilds itself over and over again throughout your lifetime. In fact, every 7 to 10 years, nearly every part of your body is regenerated, but in order to perform this amazing feat your body needs certain raw materials and nutrients.

Research has discovered and identified about 50 of these essential factors that must come from our environment.[1] Approximately 45 of them are nutrients. These essential nutrients include 20 or 21 minerals, 13 vitamins, 8 amino acids, and 2 fatty acids. They also include sources of energy from fats, protein, and carbohydrates, and invaluable elements found in water, oxygen, and light.

WATER

The most important nutrient your body needs above all others is water. Without a steady supply of water your body cannot survive longer than 3 days. Since it is the largest component of your body, used in almost every cell for all the chemical reactions and processes they perform every day, it is essential that you consume the freshest, cleanest water available, free of chemical poisons, biological toxins, and any other type of harmful products, which includes hundreds and in some places even thousands of ingredients leaching into our water supply some added by local, regional, state, and/or federal water agencies. These unnatural substances can do tremendous harm to your entire body, especially your skin, kidneys, liver, digestive system, and brain.

An easy way to clean the water you drink is to filter toxins out of it with an assortment of different filter products. I recommend a good reverse osmosis system or a similar filter for the water you use for drinking and cooking.

Some people do not consider water to be an essential part of their daily diet but water is extremely important for every chemical and biological process in your body's cells. Some researchers believe that most diseases are at least partly caused by a lack of water. Your body functions best when you drink an adequate amount of fluids, including water, that correspond with your body weight, gender, age, and activity level. Generally speaking, most medical professionals and nutritionists agree that approximately 64 ounces of water (the equivalent of 8 glasses) should be consumed daily, in whatever individual amounts suit you best. We must also calculate the amount of water we consume in other drinks and in some foods. I suggest you consult a nutritionist to gather more detailed information that will correlate with your specific diet.

As you will discover in the next chapter when we discuss quantum energy, water is not just simply H_2O. It has memory and holds energy, which can be changed from bad to good with prayer and intention, which can help make the water change into a product your body can use in a positive way, free of harm.

FATS, SUGARS, AND PROTEINS

All three of these nutrients are necessary for your body to function and important to consume wisely for optimal health.

Fats

As we discovered in chapter 1, one of the common denominators linking healthy societies is the availability and use of a good source of oils and fats. Dr. Weston Price, a dentist and researcher who focused on finding the cause of cavities and gum disease during the 1930s and 1940s, found that every thriving society from all different parts of the world had access to good sources of natural oils or fats. Residents of the Pacific Islands used palm oil, Arctic folks used animal fats, and communities in Africa and Asia profited from a mixture of raw milk and vegetable oils. What linked these societies together was their use of fresh, raw fat sources for the oils in their diets. None of them were cooked, super-heated or destroyed, as we see all too often in the way we use oils and fats in our modern Western societies. None of them destroyed the God-given natural benefits or chemical structures of these fats by pasteurizing or homogenizing their oils, as we often do in our mass-produced consumer society. All the fats Dr. Price researched were free of the added chemical hormones or preservatives we find now in man-made products in most grocery stores.[2]

Your body takes in raw, clean fats and oils and changes them into many different products and structures in your body. Fats are used to build the cell wall of every cell in your body. They are needed to maintain your body's chemical and digestive balance, produce necessary hormones and to fight chronic inflammation, which causes heart disease, cancer, dementia, and degenerative diseases.

We need two essential fatty acids in our diet—LA and LNA—that the body cannot make itself and must come from your food. They are changed in the body to other structures that can be used for energy, production of hormones, building cells, fighting pain, and the prevention and treatment of most degenerative diseases.[3]

Societies with a fresh, raw source of good oils do not suffer from the chronic illnesses of "civilized society." These good fats help protect and maintain balance in the body and prevent disease. We will learn later about the Zone diet, created by Dr. Barry Sears, which explains how these oils help your body maintain optimal health. For example, he recommends 2.5 grams a day of EPA/DHA oils. The easiest way to achieve this is to include fish oil, cod liver oil, or olive oil with your meals, preferably uncooked, lightly cooked or in a supplement form, such as capsules or liquids. I put these oils in my breakfast smoothie and take capsules of fish oil with meals.[4]

Oils put on foods after cooking work well, too, and some oils are more stable than others during low-heat cooking. Look for fresh, unprocessed oils, such as cold pressed extra virgin olive oil, high-dose fish oil capsules, and cod liver oil liquid. These oils are your best way to control silent inflammation in your body and stay in balance.

Certain populations and individuals cannot tolerate plant oils due to a genetic mutation that keeps them from metabolizing these fats. Population affected might include some West Coast natives, North Americans, Intuits, Orientals, Norwegian (like me), and Welsh/Irish people. These people traditionally use fish oils instead from a source of coldwater fish as a staple of their diets.[5]

For a detailed explanation of everything you could possibly want to know about oils and fats I suggest a book by Udo Erasmus, called *Fats That Heal, Fats That Kill*. He describes the biology of fats and oils and presents the most current information on healthy fats that prevent and undo "irreversible" degenerative diseases, such as heart disease, cancer, type II diabetes, arthritis, obesity, and many other conditions.[6]

Unfortunately, these extremely important keys to optimal health and preventing disease are almost completely forgotten in the Standard American Diet (SAD) of civilized society, which still includes cooked, processed, and chemically altered fats in its recommended diet. These can cause disease and even kill vulnerable people. Instead, eating fresh, raw, natural fats can heal and keep you in balance.

Protein

Proteins make up about 75 percent of the solid part of the body. In order to make and maintain these structures, you need to get protein from the foods you eat. The two major sources of protein are animal protein and plant protein.[7]

Your body takes in protein and breaks it apart into amino acids. Each protein is a chain of smaller amino acids glued together in a specific shape. There are about 150 different amino acids and we can make most of them inside our own bodies when we need them. However, we cannot make approximately 22 of these amino acids so they need to be supplied by the foods we eat. These essential amino acids are listed here.

ESSENTIAL AMINO ACIDS

Alanine, Arginine, Asparagine, Aspartic acid, Carnitine, Cystine and Cysteine, Glutamic acid and Glutamine, Glycine, Histidine, Leucine, Lysine, Methionine, Ornithine, Phenylalanine, Proline, Taurine, Threonine, Tryptophan, and Tyrosine.[8]

Some of these amino acids have been linked to specific illnesses and are of great importance in the prevention and reversal of some chronic illnesses. For example, research shows that lysine and proline are extremely important in the prevention of heart disease. Arginine is associated with less cavities and keeping a strong immune system. Cysteine, methionine, and taurine are all powerful sulfur-based amino acids that are used for detoxification of the body. Others are used for brain function, organ function, blood sugar regulation, collagen formation, fat metabolism, blood pressure control, and many other functions in the body.[9]

Some food sources provide complete proteins, meaning these proteins have all essential amino acids in one food. Complete proteins are eggs, meat, poultry, fish, and milk products. Some grains come very close to having a complete list of amino acids in them, including teff, amaranth, and spelt.

Most vegetable proteins do not contain all these amino acids in one food and have to be combined with others to get all of the amino acid building blocks. Most societies around the world have gotten over this by combining different plant sources to complement each other. Together, they contain the amino acids we need to maintain optimal health and vitality.

For example, Mexico combines rice, beans, and tortillas in many dishes. Middle Easterners mix chickpeas and bulgur wheat. Asians use tofu and rice. East Indians combine dahl (split peas or mung beans) and rice. These combinations can provide your body with all essential amino acids, so it can make and maintain these proteins.[10]

We don't need as much protein each day as is often suggested here in America. In fact, many people in our "civilized" society consume too much protein. The body needs 30 percent of its calories from protein to be in balance. This translates to approximately three ounces of low-fat protein a day for average-sized women and four ounces for men. We should prefer low-fat sources because the more fat in your protein the higher the arachidonic acid levels, which often triggers chronic inflammation and pain.[11]

If you eat more than this recommended amount of protein the extra protein will be changed into carbohydrates or fat for storage. This excess protein turns into fat storage and is the leading cause of obesity today in America.[12]

What do the proteins I eat have to do with my teeth and gums?

Great question! Your teeth are mainly inorganic minerals with some organic proteins holding the minerals together. But your gums are mostly made of fats and proteins. If you are low in fats and proteins your gums will be weak and unable to fight off invaders and infection. Fats and proteins are used to make new gums and repair injured gums. They are necessary for your immune system and the detoxification systems in your mouth and whole body.

For example, lysine, combined with a coenzyme, is used to fend off viruses and heal herpes lesions. As previously mentioned, the more arginine (soy, seafood, nuts, and seeds) you have in your diet the fewer cavities you will experience. The albumin protein is one of the highest antioxidants in your body, which fights inflammation and free radical damage.[13]

Let's not forget to discuss milk, which is a complete protein and the perfect natural food for babies and calves. Breast milk, raw milk, and raw dairy products, free of chemical poisons, can be useful as a fat and protein source. These raw, natural milk, and dairy products are the common denominator in some of the healthiest groups of people around the world.

Milk that has been processed, homogenized, and filled with chemicals is not the best food for humans, especially babies. Pasteurization heats up milk's fats and proteins to very high temperatures, which denatures (destroys) the food into an unnatural product that the body cannot use.

Hormones found in processed milk have been linked to hormone imbalances, depression, cancer, juvenile diabetes, cataracts, immune system deficiencies, allergies, and other conditions.

Although milk has some calcium in it, it contains far too much phosphorus and actually depletes the calcium in the body as it processes this extra phosphorus and complex protein. Unless you are using raw dairy products for fats and protein sources, it would be best to avoid any processed dairy products.[14]

Carbohydrates

We need these simple and complex sugars in our diet, mainly to fuel the body and to add some fiber, vitamins, minerals, and water.

Simple carbohydrates are considered sugary food because of its simple sugar structure, which can be easily broken down and used in your bloodstream. Sugar, honey, syrup, and candy are some of the simple sugars.

Complex carbohydrates are complex sugar structures that are not usually broken down easily in the blood. These include fruits, vegetables, starches, pastas, breads, potatoes, and rice.[15]

A commonly held belief for a long time was that natural, raw complex carbohydrates were better for you than simple carbohydrates. But new research started to measure the effect that different carbohydrates have on the blood and the results were surprising. It was found that some simple carbohydrates enter the bloodstream as glucose at a much slower rate than complex carbohydrates. In fact, *all* sugars and carbohydrates are broken down in the body into simple sugars, such as glucose and fructose.[16]

Grains and starches are composed of long strings of 100 percent glucose, held together by weak bonds, which break easily, causing the food containing glucose entering the bloodstream to rapidly increase the body's insulin response.

Vegetables (30 percent fructose) and fruits (70 percent fructose) are rapidly absorbed but slowly converted into glucose in the liver. Therefore, foods in the form of fructose will actually be converted into glucose slower than complex carbohydrates that are already 100 percent glucose (grains and starches).

This is why complex carbohydrates, such as rice cakes and potatoes, have a faster rate of absorption/glycemic load than sugar (half fructose, half glucose) or honey, which is 100 percent fructose.[17]

The glycemic load is a combination of how fast a food is absorbed and the amount of carbohydrate that is in the food. Foods high on the glycemic load have been linked to obesity, diabetes, and heart attacks. This is because of the silent chronic inflammation that the carbohydrates cause in your body.

VITAMINS

Vitamins are micronutrients, meaning they are only necessary in small amounts. They regulate how good your body's system will work and are used in every cell of your body. They are found in our food and drink, and some, like Vitamin D, are manufactured in our own bodies.

If your body becomes low in certain vitamins it can make you become susceptible to a wide variety of conditions and diseases, such of which are listed here. The following list includes diseases and/or conditions and the corresponding vitamin deficiency, which may cause those health issues.[18]

Table 3.1. Symptoms of Vitamin Deficiency

Health Issue	Vitamin Deficiency
Appetite loss	A, B1, C, biotin
Cholesterol high	B complex, B3, inositol, choline
Fatigue	A, B complex, PABA, C, D
High Blood pressure	Choline
Memory loss	B1, choline
Mouth sores	B2, B6, lysine
Muscle cramps	B1, B6, biotin, D, E, K
Skin problems	A, B complex, inositol
Slow healing	A, C
Soft teeth and bones	D

Severe vitamin deficiencies can be life threatening. The more we cook, process, and change the foods we eat, the more vitamins and minerals we take out of the food we rely on to give us what we need to achieve and maintain optimal health and vitality.

Do you remember the story of sailors and scurvy from the previous chapter? It demonstrates the acute danger a vitamin deficiency can cause. We know that humans, guinea pigs, and rhesus monkeys are the only species that cannot make their own vitamin C through a natural process within the body. Cats, dogs, and other animals manufacture all the vitamin C they need, but we need to supply our bodies with vitamin C from the foods we eat and/or supplements.

In the past, fruits and vegetables were our main source of vitamin C. With the manipulation of our fruits and vegetables by genetic mutations, processing, and spraying with chemicals, our foods do not contain the same amount of vitamin C anymore, which means that if you want to get an adequate level of vitamin C from the oranges currently available on commercial markets you will have to eat an entire box of oranges in order to get the vitamin C you need each day.

Your gums need 3,000 to 5,000 mg of vitamin C a day to be healthy and able to repair tissues, fight off invaders, and keep from bleeding. As we saw in the past with those sailors at sea, if you don't get enough vitamin C your gums will also start to bleed.[19]

Gums need certain nutrients to build and repair. They require vitamin C, CoQ10, vitamin B complex, vitamin D, along with a good source of protein and nutrients.

Vitamin D

Vitamin D has taken on new life as an extremely important vitamin for the body's protection and prevention of disease. Although we have known that vitamin D, calcium, and boron are essential for our bones and teeth, we know now that vitamin D has other important functions, for example, making the glue that holds your cells together. Vitamin D is necessary to form a strong bond between every one of your body's cells.

When you are vitamin D deficient you cannot keep the strong bond between cells, allowing bad bugs to invade and leak into the body. This weakens the integrity of the body and can allow cancer to invade, infections to spread, and tissues to break down.

High levels of vitamin D reduce the risk of breast cancer and prostate cancer, and one study shows vitamin D decreasing the rate of all cancers by 77 percent.[20]

MINERALS

Minerals are ionic or charged forms of metal and other elements. They are simple in structure, and like vitamins they are used together with other minerals, vitamins, and macronutrients to perform their function in the body.

Major minerals are needed in large amounts, such as calcium, magnesium, phosphorus, sodium, and potassium. Minor or trace minerals are needed but only in small amounts.

Calcium, phosphorus, and boron are needed to build strong bones and teeth, muscles, and to keep the heart healthy. Zinc is needed for taste, smell, brain function, prostate and hormone function, and many other uses. Magnesium is used to relax muscles, regulate the heart, and control bowel function.[21]

Minerals can also interplay and interfere with each other. For example, raising the phosphorus level in our SAD diet (red meat, red wine, and processed foods) uses up the magnesium in the body and can cause muscle cramps and heart palpitations.[22]

Most minerals have a hard time crossing into the blood stream from the GI tract and need to be transported by chelators, which are better absorbed by the body. When taking micro minerals look for chelated or dipeptide chelated minerals for better absorption.[23]

We can no longer get enough vitamins and minerals from our foods alone. We need 13 vitamins and 20 different minerals to maintain optimal health and vitality. Look for a good complimentary or alternative medical practitioner to help you find and evaluate the vitamins and minerals in your body and to determine what you need to supplement for your individual balance.

As a rule, vitamins are better absorbed with meals and minerals are better absorbed on an empty stomach. Your body needs to eat and absorb minerals to build strong teeth and bone. They can't just be any type of minerals. If you take, for example calcium carbonate, a far less absorbable type of mineral, it passes right through the body without ever being absorbed. If you take the less absorbable minerals, you are wasting your money, since these are far more useless to the body.

Calcium and magnesium that are chelated (bound together) with an amino acid are far more absorbable by the body and useful for building blocks. They can pass into the body from your GI tract and be used to build strong teeth and bones.

I take a few supplements listed below for the conditions I have. Different people absorb different vitamins and minerals differently so you need to make sure you get the right type of vitamins and minerals that your body can use. You will have a unique list of things that you need to supplement.

There are easy tests for you to take at home for Omega 3 oils, vitamin C, vitamin D, zinc, and niacin. Most good alternative health care practitioners can also perform these and other tests for you. Blood tests check levels of vitamins and minerals, except magnesium. Testing magnesium is different because 98 percent of all your magnesium is inside your cells, not running around in your bloodstream or urine. You can test for magnesium if you look inside the cell, which you can do with an intracellular test for magnesium by a company called Exatest. It effectively and accurately measures the magnesium you are getting and absorbing.

More information on magnesium and other minerals in the body is available from a number of sources but for now here is a list of vitamins and minerals that your teeth and gums need to be strong and healthy.[24]

ESSENTIAL VITAMINS AND MINERALS

The essential vitamins are: A, D, E, K, C, Bioflavonoids, B1, B2, B3, B5, B6, B12, B15, B17, Folic acid, Biotin, PABA, Inositol, Choline, and CoQ10.

The essential minerals are: Calcium, Chloride, Chromium, Cobalt, Copper, Iodine, Iron, Lithium, Magnesium, Manganese, Molybdenum, Phosphorus, Potassium, Selenium, Sodium, Sulfur, Vanadium, and Zinc.

RECOMMENDED DIETS

Many of my patients ask me to pick the correct diet for them or want a second opinion on what foods to eat. Everyone is individual and has many conditions that affect their nutritional needs. Since I am not an M.D. or N.D. and not a licensed dietician or nutritionist, I can only provide some insight, based on years of my own research and practice, how I would choose a diet and where I would go for advice.

Let's begin with Carolyn Mein and the Body Type diet. She teaches that there are 25 different body types based on your dominant organs. Inspired by Chinese body type studies, she teaches that an individual needs to determine what body he or she has and then figure out a diet that supports them best.[25]

I am a Thalamus body type, which means there are foods that support me and foods that are bad for me. I take this list and go to the Zone Anti-inflammatory diet and remove foods with a high glycemic load and use mostly low glycemic foods. The Anti-inflammatory Zone diet keeps your body in a balanced state so it can run smoothly and remain disease free.[26]

I would consult with Ed Group and his extensive knowledge of foods, cycles of the body's functions, and detox to double check what kinds of foods to eat and at what time of the day. His books and website are full of helpful advice that goes further beyond foods to include green and healthy living in all areas. He offers extensive detox programs, fasting protocols, and clean and healthy living resources.[27]

I believe one thing is more important than the physical foods you eat and drink, and that is the energy of the nutrients we consume. Everything that goes into your mouth—food, drink, and supplements—should be blessed and prayed over so they can be helpful to your body and have no bad effects. We will explain this process in Part III of this book.

A DEEPER DIVE INTO OUR DIET

In order to fully appreciate the need for a healthy diet, we should also describe the physics of the body and how it is all connected. Dr. Price's studies can help us with that, as we can see from the changes in people's health when some primitive and isolated people left their communities and went out into the world. He studied groups of people that moved into the modern civilization and documented the changes in their health, including the start of cavities and gum disease that were not there before.

For example, Dr. Price noted the teeth of the Eskimos, whose teeth were often worn nearly to the gum line and yet their gum tissue had not receded. Many of these primitive groups were practically free from the affliction we know now as pyorrhea or gingivitis. In the light of our new knowledge, pyorrhea is largely a nutritional problem. While nutrition alone will not often be adequate for correcting it, practically no treatment will be completely adequate without reinforcing proper nutrition, as it is always a contributing factor.[28]

Dr. Price theorized that there must be some food substance that is not adequately provided in modern nutrition, perhaps owing to some fundamental change in quantity, preparation, or selection of the substance. From observing skeletal structures, he deduced that people from primitive societies obtained a substance that a modern generation does not have. His book presents evidence for the "activator X" substance he labeled as this missing food substance. He theorized it was not one of the recognized vitamins because he ruled them out one by one, but a substance belonging in the fat-soluble group.

His data stated that the "activator X" had the following characteristics:

1. It played an essential role in the maximum utilization of bodybuilding minerals and tissues.

2. It was present in the butterfat of milk of mammals, the eyes of fishes, and the organ and fats of animals.
3. It is synthesized by the mammary glands and plays an important role in infant growth and also in reproduction.[29]

Diet is a good place to start living healthier. We will describe the importance of other influences such as: pH levels, Ca/PO4 ratio, water, different bacteria we have in our bodies, essential oils and herbs, levels of oxidative stress, antioxidants, and many other factors.

When man started to refine sugar, he changed the natural sugars and God-made raw foods into something far more destructive and dangerous. When man removed the natural sugar beet, sugar cane, fruit, and honey from whole foods through cooking and processing, he dramatically changed the substance and the effect they have on the body.

BEWARE THE ACID ATTACK!

Our bodies metabolize simple and complex carbohydrates differently. For example, when one eats a carrot the sugar it contains, combined with its fiber, minerals, and vitamins, is not broken down by the bacteria in your mouth fast enough to cause cavities. It would take hours and days for the bacteria to break down these complex carbohydrates and natural sugars into the acids that eat away your teeth.

This is why natural foods, such as carrots, apples, broccoli, nuts, and seeds can make excellent snacks. Later we will share tips on the best snack foods for your teeth and a list of foods that can be eaten between meals without worrying about your teeth or gums. This includes natural snacks, foods, and even candies that can fight cavities and are excellent snack foods at any time of the day because they are all meant to avoid feeding the bad bacteria, which prevents them from turning sugar into acid. In fact, some of them actively kill the bacteria that cause cavities and gum disease.

Here is the dental problem with processed and refined simple sugars:

Bad bacteria change the sugar into acid very quickly.

Almost immediately after you eat or drink a simple sugar the cavity bugs in your mouth change the sugar in your mouth to acid, which starts to dissolve your teeth until your own saliva can dilute the acid in about 20 minutes.

Therefore, after eating or drinking a simple sugar product, your mouth has to endure a *20-minute acid attack*. We will teach you ways to avoid this acid attack even when you eat simple sugars.

It's easy to see why the safer snacks that can take hours or days to be broken down can be safely cleaned off the teeth before the acid attack. The bacteria don't have time to destroy the teeth when safer snack foods are chosen and if the teeth are effectively cleaned before they have a chance to make the acid.

WHAT ABOUT GLUTEN?

A lot of attention is being paid to gluten these days primarily because of its perceived effect on our digestion. While this is true for some people, there are other equally important reasons for *everyone* to pay attention to their consumption of gluten.

Refined flours and pastas, which are full of gluten, play a big role in causing dental disease. Although breads and pastas are not simple sugars, they can do as much damage as simple sugars. In fact, they can be worse than a simple sugar that only stays in the mouth for a few minutes.

Even though these are more complex carbohydrates (sugars), they contain a sticky substance called *gluten* that holds them together, and in the case of bread, for example, what holds the wheat and other substances together also sticks to your teeth for a long time. If you are eating refined white flour in a piece of bread or a muffin or cake, the gluten can stay there for days and weeks if not cleaned by you. This stickiness allows bad bacteria to break down more complex sugars into acid and starts to dissolve your teeth.

In fact, this is how some of the cavity research for cavities is performed. Small amounts of moist bread are attached to the side of the teeth of experimental animals and left for weeks. After two to three weeks on the tooth, the bacteria change the sugars to acid and start a white spot on the tooth, which is the beginning of a cavity.

This same process happens when we eat refined grains and do not effectively clean between the teeth and in the deep grooves or around past fillings and crowns. This is why you need to thoroughly clean your teeth after you have consumed *any* type of solid or liquid carbohydrates. The simple sugars make acid immediately and the more complex sugars cause cavities after days and weeks.

For example, when you combine these sugars in a peanut butter and jelly sandwich for lunch at school, the simple sugars added to make the jelly immediately start to eat away at the teeth and the sticky bread stays on the teeth all day to cause further acid destruction. Later, we will present effective ways to create a great lunch for your kids and how to never let bugs start cavities. For now, just remember this:

Simple sugars eat the teeth for 20 minutes and complex carbohydrates can be dangerous if left on the teeth and not cleaned off immediately.

I get a lot of patients that obsess about a tiny ingredient in some product or food. They miss the overriding concept of holistic health; that we have to look at the whole body not just one tiny part.

NUTRITION AND YOUR IMMUNE SYSTEM

Maintaining balance in the inner workings of our body is the most important thing we can do—even more significant than tooth brushing, mouth rinses, flossing, and even the oral irrigator, and cleanings at the dentist!

The dietary guidelines introduced here are crucial to the health of the rest of the body and directly influence your oral health. Many dental and medical websites, lectures, researchers, and scientists explain numerous products, foods, dietary, and lifestyle changes that can give you powerful tools to kill bad bugs, assist good bugs, heal tissue, build up your defenses, and stay healthy and in balance.

Jonathan Wright, M.D. delivered a lecture at the International Association of Oral Medicine and Toxicology's March 2003 convention. I listened to him speak about nutrition and oral health, specifically about preventing cavities and gum disease, bone loss, and staying healthy.

For cavity prevention he, like many dentists, recommended eliminating refined sugar and refined carbohydrates, soft drinks, and minimizing fruit juices. He recommended chewing xylitol gum or mints three to four times a day and suggested adding strontium, vitamin K, and pyridoxine supplements to one's diet to help keep the body's immune system strong.

For gum disease prevention he recommended supplementing the diet with CQ10, folic acid, calcium, and vitamins C and E. For prevention of bone loss he recommended supplements to the diet of Betaine hydrochloride with pepsin, calcium, magnesium, strontium, vitamins D and K, and Ipriflavone. He also recommended limiting milk, choosing tea over coffee, moderating protein intake, emphasizing vegetables and fruits, and avoiding gluten, fluoride, lead, and heavy metals.

Here is a concise list of his recommendations:

DR. WRIGHT'S RECOMMENDATIONS

Caries prevention:

1. Eliminate sugar, refined carbohydrates, and soft drinks, and minimize fruit juices.
2. Use Xylitol chewing gum or mints 3x/day.
3. Take strontium (200 to 300 mg/day for adults, 50 to 200 mg/day for children).
4. Use vitamin K dental spray with toothpaste 2x/day.
5. Use pyridoxine (10 to 50 mg/day).

Periodontal disease prevention:

1. Take CoQ10 30 mg/twice a day.
2. Use a folic acid oral rinse 2x/day.
3. Take calcium (1 gram/day with magnesium 300 to 400 mg/day).
4. Take vitamin C (1 gram/twice a day).
5. Take vitamin E (400 to 800 IU/day).[30]

These are certainly a good start and nice to hear from a traditional doctor. Dental and medical research continues to expand and we are further refining the supplements we need and don't get from our foods.

I provide my patients with a list of recommended supplements for healthy teeth and gums. It's been developed from a variety of sound scientific research and I am pleased to include it here to help you keep your body in balance.

Table 3.2. Recommended Supplements for Healthy Gums

Supplement	Daily Dosage	Actions/Benefits
Vitamin C	3,000 mg– 5,000 mg	Antioxidant, body repair; slows aging; builds collagen, bones, and teeth; scurvy, gingivitis, ulcers if deficient
Coenzyme Q10	60 mg	Similar to Vit. E but more powerful, stimulates immune system, oxygenates tissue, heals gum tissue
Omega 3 fatty acids	EPA 2500 mg DHA 2500 mg	Decreases inflammation in gum tissues
Vitamin A	4000 IU-females

5000 IU-males | Increases cytokine production which stimulates host resistance, controls cell growth and development |
Calcium	1000 mg– 1500 mg	Builds strong teeth, jaws, and bone, used for muscle contraction, and gum tissue
Magnesium	600 mg	Bone, carbohydrate, and mineral metabolism, energy in the cell, mineral transport
Folic acid	800 mcg	DNA synthesis, cell growth, and tissue keratinization
Niacin	420 mg	Pellagra—gingivitis, gum ulcers if lacking
Riboflavin	34 mg	Glossitis, angular cheilosis if lacking, helps in tissue oxidation
Vitamin D	2000IU	Aids in adsorbing Ca, Phos., and Mg, builds bone from cartilage
Strontium	200 mg	Aids in bone and teeth repair
Selenium	200 mcg	Decreases inflammation, anti-oxidant
Zinc	35 mg	Host resistance, healing and decreases inflammation

REBUILDING YOUR TEETH WITH GOOD NUTRITION

As we mentioned, there are groups of people around the world that don't have access to toothbrushes, toothpastes, mouth rinse, or dentists. They don't have tooth decay or gum disease. This is because their diet, the most important physical factor, is absolutely healthy, and it goes to show that diet and a healthy immune system, including the ratio of good bugs and bad bugs, are far more important than the toothpaste you use.

I hear about many patients using inferior toothpastes who are disease-free. That's because they have great diets and have achieved balance in their lives. The body needs certain raw materials to create the building blocks of the teeth and gums and in many cases, to repair them, as well.

All of the communities Dr. Price documented used organic, local, raw foods, rich in good fats, calcium, and phosphate. They ate alkaline foods and rarely cooked them. Their bodies could easily metabolize these naturally, unaltered, uncooked, unprocessed foods, allowing them to prosper and live with optimal vitality.

FOODS AND pH LEVELS AND YOUR BODY

We use some of the same foods today for our meals and safe snacks. These include raw dairy products (raw milk, cream, cheeses, and butter), nuts and seeds, soy, and fish and high arginine foods. Snacks of cacao chocolate, hard cheeses, and raw fruits and vegetables can be powerful sources of the building blocks that your body needs to rebuild, repair, and strengthen your teeth and gums.[31]

Let's look at some of the common snacks and soft drinks that are available and popular with kids and adults and see if they are all they're cracked up top be. For example, we often hear through spirited advertising campaigns that sport drinks are healthy but is that really true? We must determine their sugar content and look at the pH levels and corrosive potential these products have on your teeth.

The pH (potential of Hydrogen) level of your body is extremely important. It is a measure of acidity or alkalinity of water-soluble substances and is measured on a scale of 1 to 14, with 7 as the middle or neutral point—meaning values below seven indicate acidity with one being the most acidic. Alkaline foods and snacks help to maintain a neutral pH in the mouth. Stay away from acidic foods and snacks in between meals when the teeth need to rebuild.

Table 3.3.   **Food Acid and Sports Drink**

Drink/Food	pH	Dissolving Power	Erosion
Water	7.28	0.02	low
Whole milk	6.69	0.1	low
Natural cheese	5.01	0.5	medium
Seedless raisins	3.98	2.59	high
Dried apricots	3.87	2.49	high
Red Bull	3.32		high
Grapefruit juice	3.2	9.3	highest
Apple juice	3.2	4.5	very high
Gatorade	2.95		high
Powerade	2.78		high
Cola	2.5	0.7	medium

Source: Noble, Warden H., DDS, MS, MSED, et al., *"Sports Drinks and Dental Erosion," JADA,* Vol. 39, no. 4, April 2011, 233–34.

After a hard workout or sports event you go to replenish your body's electrolytes and the loss of water you sweated out. You grab a Red Bull (pH = 3.32), a Gatorade (pH = 2.95), or PowerAde (pH = 2.78). You avoid any cola products (pH = 2–4) because they are known to be too acidic and dehydrating.[32]

All four of these sports drinks are below the 4.5 pH level that is the borderline to a pH that destroys your teeth. Any of these drinks will dissolve your teeth quickly and if in contact with your teeth for a long time (sipping on a drink for a period of time) they will destroy your tooth's enamel.

The fruit juices: orange juice (pH = 3.8), apple juice (pH = 3.2), and grapefruit juice (pH = 3.2) are not any better at keeping your mouth in a healthy pH balance. All three have high erosion potential to destroy your teeth. If you use these remember to keep them off the teeth for extended periods of time. Drink the whole amount at one time, rinse with plain water right away, or even better brush your teeth after drinking them. Use a straw to avoid the contact with your teeth as much as possible.[33]

Cool water at a pH of about 7.28 is usually the best drink to refresh. Electrolytes can be added with Emergen-C powder as a powerful boost.

There is one drink that has the potential to help build the teeth, which plain water cannot do. This product is root beer. Many studies have been performed to evaluate the pH and erosive properties of all the popular drinks. Root beer always comes out with the least erosive potential. It outperforms even water. By avoiding erosion, your teeth have time to rebuild. The best would be root beer without caffeine and sweetened with stevia instead of sugar.

A second good option is cool flavored water (Kool-Aid) made with stevia, not sugar and with added Emergen-C electrolytes. This can refresh, rejuvenate, and avoid the erosion of your teeth after a hard workout.

FINAL THOUGHTS

The organic tissue parts of your gums and bones are made up of proteins, fats, and carbohydrates. The inorganic parts of your teeth and bones are made up from the vitamins and minerals you eat. Gum cells and tissue need high quality protein and good fats to make healthy cell walls, tissue, and organs.

The teeth and gums also need a healthy body (environment) to grow, repair, and maintain optimal health. This means things like your Ca/PO4 ratio, pH, level of chronic inflammation, oxidative stress, antioxidant levels, and quality of water.[34]

Like vitamins, all minerals are necessary and many of them work together with other minerals, vitamins, and macronutrients (foods) for your benefit.

The balance between them is often more important than the presence of an absolute amount.

For example, calcium, in combination with phosphorus, is important for strong bones and healthy teeth. The calcium/phosphorus ratio in a healthy body must be in a range of 2.5 to 1. If you get too much calcium, the excess can contribute to arthritis, bone spurs, calcium deposits in the arteries, kidney stones, and gall stones. If the phosphorus is too high, as can happen when eating fish, meat, dairy, cheeses, or soft drinks (with phosphoric acid), then the body may pull out calcium from your bones and teeth to maintain the ideal balance.

Balancing vitamins, minerals, and foods is the key to optimal health and vitality.

Unfortunately, most dentists rarely talk about these important things and they miss out on providing their patients with wholesome, holistic care. These conditions, and the way you take care of yourself through a nutritional perspective, regulate the fundamental environment of your body. They are far more important than worrying about the specific ingredients in your toothpaste or if you floss.

Once again, you are what you eat, and choosing the right foods and supplements will keep you (and your teeth and gums) healthy and enjoying the gift of good meals.

4

Chakras, Meridians, and the Heart: How Matter and Energy Affect Your Oral Health

This chapter could also be titled "Your Teeth and Quantum Physics" because it presents a simple explanation of selected quantum physics principles that have the potential to be used to improve your immune system, heal from imbalances, strengthen your body defenses, and achieve and maintain optimal health and vitality.

Quantum physics is now beginning to describe and document this healing universe with the same descriptions and definitions that have been used for centuries by Aborigines, Native Americans, and mystics from all corners of the world.[1]

This ancient form of science, combined with a seasoned spirituality, is telling us we are all one and that we are living within the same energy field (e = mc^2). Since we all are connected, we affect each other. This "entanglement" is the result of an ultimate being, known in quantum physics circles as the Zero Point Field.[2]

Many people believe we are sparks emanating from the Divine Spark and co-creators of our lives through downward causation. Whatever your religious inclinations may be, the study of physics and energy is an important scientific element to consider when it comes to our health.

The healing energy of pets and the grounding energy of nature show that everything is connected, and we only need to observe an expanded view of the body's chakras, meridian system, and heart influence to understand how these forces affect us.

Higher and faster energy can change your physical world and the universe around you. For example, water crystals can change their properties through the influence of love and gratitude. We also see this demonstrated through prayer and intention, both of which can physically change your food and drink—and your teeth and gums.

PHYSICS AND THE WORLD

I remember during my grade school years being fascinated with an educational movie at school called *The Powers of 10*. It was a visual tour of our universe, starting with a close-up view of people in a park before the camera pulled out to show more people in the entire park, then quickly expanded its view to reveal a city, state, and country perspective before moving rapidly into space, providing a view of the earth, the planets, our solar system, universe, and beyond.

Even at an early age I was fascinated with this expanded view of our world. I wondered how all of this might affect us here on earth and this led to my exploring these possibilities as a dentist. This process, trying to understand the concepts of physics and cosmic energy, can be daunting and confusing. For now, let's focus on the simple concepts that directly affect our dental health.

That begins with a basic view of the world of physics, which is man's attempt to explain how our world works. The first person to make his mark in this field was a man named Newton. He came up with a novel concept of gravity, which tried to explain how the world works through four main forces—strong, weak, gravitational, and electromagnetic. Every reaction in chemistry, biology, and biochemistry could be calculated with these forces. Physics was developing as the basic science that could explain all the natural sciences and how the world works.

In biology, each part of the body was broken down into their separate function and parts in order to explain them. Each organ's chemistry and biochemistry was explained by breaking the function into chemical reactions. The body and medical diagnosis and treatments broke up the body into individual parts in order to explain the whole. The scientists and doctors were trying to explain how our bodies worked. Individual studies in petri dishes of corresponding chemical reactions in the body were studied, classified, and analyzed.

This breakdown of the body helped scientists understand its functions. As a result, doctors eventually began to specialize in certain parts of the body and neglected the rest of it, which produced generations of experts who knew everything about your eyes, ears, nose, throat, GI tract, lungs, heart, feet, hands, internal organs, brain, skin, and mouth, but little about the rest of the body and how it interacted with other parts as a whole, not to mention the effects of emotion and spirituality.

Scientists realized that there were still parts of the world and unexplained events that affect the body and that these could not be explained by examining parts of the whole body. Scientists dug deeper for answers, breaking chemicals down into individual DNA, and some have gone even further into the structure of these particles and have found they are made up of things like quarks and mesons.

QUANTUM PHYSICS

This science is man's attempt to explain how the world works by establishing a unifying theory that explains everything in the universe. Scientists have discovered some amazing clues that explain many things more accurately then Newtonian physics could, theories and activities that have baffled us for a long time. These scientists are also using some unusual terms and concepts to describe universal properties and laws—poetic imagery that describes the basic building blocks of the world we live in.[3]

They are seeing how things separated by great distances affect each other without any known connections. They are seeing people's belief and emotions affect the physical world around them. They are starting to explain how amazing, miraculous things can happen with this new theory, and are even starting to develop proof that a personal God exists. It is an amazing field of study and we provide references in the back of this book so you can pursue this further if you wish.

One of the most famous ideas in quantum physics is Einstein's formula: $e = mc^2$. We've all learned this formula and how e equals energy, m equals mass, and c equals the speed of light. What most students fail to grasp is the profound leap in knowledge that this formula and the basic concepts that led up to it has had on our lives.

Einstein's concept explained that everything is energy and mass and that neither can be destroyed. All the energy and mass can do is turn from energy back into mass or from mass to energy.

Everything in the universe is energy. Everything you can see, feel, touch, smell, or taste contains energy particles bouncing around. The skin on your arm is not solid but particles bouncing around in a vast mostly empty space. Solid lead metal is not solid but particles bouncing around in a mostly empty space. Your teeth and gums are just particles bouncing around in mostly empty space.[4]

Quantum physics has shown how your beliefs and emotions affect the particles that make up your teeth, gums, cells, and organs. We now know all of them are affected by the energy outside of your body. We will see later how

Table 4.1. Cosmic Energy and Your Health

Newtonian Physics	Quantum Physics	God's Physics
ma = mx = F(x)	$e = mc^2$	Love
Gravity/apple	Observer changes reality	Co-creation
Logic/mathematics/predictable	Chaos/Planck constant	Free-will choice
Cause/effect	Probability/possibility	Miracles
Three dimensions	9+ dimensions	Infinite spirit
Time space/4 forces	Entanglement	Possibility
Macroscopic parts	Microscopic particle and waves	All are one

EMF energy waves, magnetic fields, laser energy, and other people's energy can affect you and your body's balance, health, and ability to fend off disease.

A holistic dentist or medical practitioner's model of health and disease tries to bring the whole body and world back into the picture. In addition to looking at the body as a whole they will show how outside influences affect your health and contribute to disease. The body works as a whole and all the parts, even far away parts of the universe, can affect your inside cells, organs, and body systems. The holistic dental model here does not just focus on the physical body but the whole person and his or her universe.

Let's take a simple concept and apply it to your health. We know that 75 percent of your body is water. Water is used in every cell for chemical and biochemical reactions. Without adequate water you would not survive longer than a few weeks. Water is vital to the health and balance of every part of your body.

Dr. Masaru Emoto (1943–2014) was an iconic Japanese scientist who exposed water to physical, emotional, and spiritual influences and analyzed it after the change. He wanted to find out if human consciousness can alter the molecular structure of water, which is conceivable if one considers the possibilities of quantum physics and the fact that our bodies are composed largely of this substance and influenced by its energy.

As part of his fascinating work, Dr. Emoto wanted to show the structure of different kinds of water and see if there was a difference. He took water from various sources, some clean, some dirty and polluted, some natural, some not, and he froze droplets of water on to slides and with a microscope he took pictures of the ice crystals that formed.[5]

His books of water crystal photos are spectacular. Some of the photos show us the beauty of pure, clean water. Other photos of polluted, dirty water tell us how our environment can destroy the structure of water.

He went further in his research to see how our society and environment have an influence on water. Do they affect the ice crystal formation? It would seem to be important especially because our own bodies are made up of so much water.

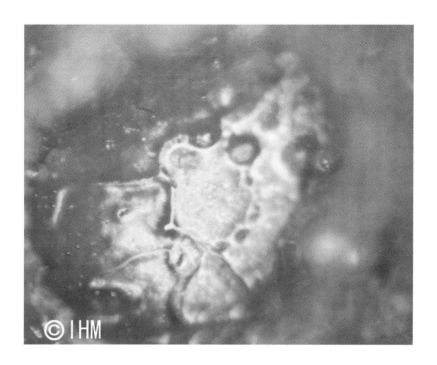

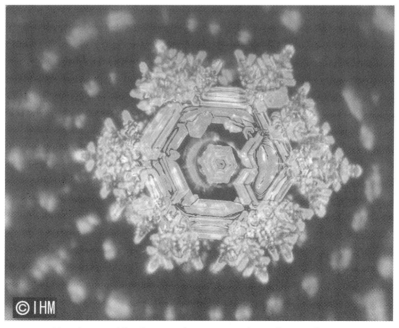

How love and forgiveness change water from chaos to beauty

Dr. Emoto found that music, sound, written and spoken words, thoughts, prayers, and blessings all had profound effects on water. Classical music, soulful music, kind words and thoughts, love and gratitude, prayers and blessings all instigated beautiful ice crystal formations.

Some hard rock music, hateful words and thoughts, fear and anger, and negative intentions changed the water, destroying its beauty, which resulted in various horrible photos of the water's destruction. It is an amazing book and field of study. Some people even put these photos up in their homes and on their office walls.

In addition to the documentary of how these different environmental factors influence water, we can take a step further and see the beginning of a new concept.

How does the environment, the music we listen to, the movies we watch, the time in front of a computer, the words we say, the thoughts we focus on all day affect our own body's water? The water our bodies are made of and relies on for millions of chemical reactions every second in our trillions of cells are affected by these influence for balance, health, and/or disease.

If we constantly listen to aggressive music, use an excessive amount of drugs and alcohol, spread hate and anger, hold on to grudges and fear for others, how does this affect our body's balance and optimal health and vitality? We can and do affect our own health. We can and do affect everyone around us. We can and do affect the water and every cell and particle in our environment. Our influence does not stop with our own body. It radiates throughout the universe.

This is the basis of applied kinesiology (AK), the muscle test diagnosis of the body's condition. This science has shown that the things we expose our bodies to can immediately affect its strength. Using muscle groups that respond to these influences, we can tell if something from the environment will make us strong or weak. For example, you can test if a package of vitamin C will make you strong and if a package of sugar will make you weak.

AK techniques are a powerful example of how something outside your body can influence your health. For example, places of high energy, such as being in church, at an inspiring concert, or on a natural beach, can potentially affect your health in a positive way. Places of low energy and fear, such as a home filled with anger and hate, an angry rally with a hateful crowd, or an environment filled with toxic behavior, can negatively affect your body and health.

Dr. David Hawkins, an iconic spiritual teacher, psychiatrist, physician, researcher, and lecturer, who developed what he calls a Map of Consciousness, has written several powerful books based on some of these concepts and the research he conducted regarding this phenomena. He begins by presenting the concept that everything is energy, including love, fear, joy, peace, anger,

MAP OF CONSCIOUSNESS®

God-view	Life-view	Level		Log	Emotion	Process
Self	Is	Enlightenment	⇑	700-1000	Ineffable	Pure Consciousness
All-Being	Perfect	Peace	⇑	600	Bliss	Illumination
One	Complete	Joy	⇑	540	Serenity	Transfiguration
Loving	Benign	Love	⇑	500	Reverence	Revelation
Wise	Meaningful	Reason	⇑	400	Understanding	Abstraction
Merciful	Harmonious	Acceptance	⇑	350	Forgiveness	Transcendence
Inspiring	Hopeful	Willingness	⇑	310	Optimism	Intention
Enabling	Satisfactory	Neutrality	⇑	250	Trust	Release
Permitting	Feasible	Courage	⇕	200	Affirmation	Empowerment
Indifferent	Demanding	Pride	⇓	175	Scorn	Inflation
Vengeful	Antagonistic	Anger	⇓	150	Hate	Aggression
Denying	Disappointing	Desire	⇓	125	Craving	Enslavement
Punitive	Frightening	Fear	⇓	100	Anxiety	Withdrawal
Disdainful	Tragic	Grief	⇓	75	Regret	Despondency
Condemning	Hopeless	Apathy	⇓	50	Despair	Abdication
Vindictive	Evil	Guilt	⇓	30	Blame	Destruction
Despising	Miserable	Shame	⇓	20	Humiliation	Elimination

Map of Consciousness

guilt, and the like, and he claims that each of these energies vibrate at different speeds. He distinguishes them by attributing arbitrary values from zero to 1,000. The way he explains this allows the reader to test the various influences of the people, places, and things in their own world.

Dr. Hawkins found that frequencies above 400 to 500 help us heal and stay balanced. Things like love, joy, and peace radiate at this healing level. We can see evidence of this healing level in a purring cat, a dog waging its tail, and a singing bird.[6]

Lower frequencies below 200 pull us down, cause disease, and take our emotions out of balance with the universe. Things like pride, anger, fear, guilt, and shame radiate at this slower frequency. We can see evidence of this in pollution, fighting, violent protest, and other bad choices and behavior.

Dr. Hawkins encourages people to learn his testing techniques and use them to measure the energy in the songs you listen to, the books you read, and the places you live. I highly recommend his books and the tests he offers.

ENERGY LEVELS AND YOUR TEETH AND GUMS

These concepts relate directly to your teeth and gums. Both areas of your mouth are susceptible to disease, and in the case of cavities and gum disease, both are host-mediated bacterial infections, triggered by bad bugs, a negative influence coming from outside your body. In fact, most of the bad bugs in your body come from being contaminated by someone around you. Most modern medicine focuses on these bugs and uses drugs, chemicals, and surgery to get rid of them. I tend to focus on you, the host, as I feel this is more important. Bad bugs are everywhere around us and we are all exposed to them, but only a few of us get the diseases they bring. That's because of you and your ability to fight off the bad bugs and repair the damage they may have started. Your body, if it is healthy and strong, fights off these invaders and keeps you at optimal health and vitality.

Our resistance does not only depend on our body. It relies on a peaceful and positive state of mind, as well, and a willing and generous spirit. For example, consider what can happen if your body is negatively influenced by slow, low energy. When you are exposed to sugar, processed foods, chaotic EMF frequencies, smoke and alcohol, pollution, fear, and anger this affects all of your cells, organs, and operational systems. Even the water of your body is affected. Slow, low energy frequencies can make us weak and susceptible to disease and bad bugs. When your defenses are down, your reparative capacity is impaired and you will not function at peak efficiency. You will get sick because when the bad bugs invade, they will thrive and cause disease to take root.

It won't matter if you brush and floss, use hand sanitizers, or cocoon yourself away from the world. Chronic inflammation and oxidative stress will increase and these two factors are more important to the health and disease of your teeth and gums.

A holistic dentist is more concerned with your whole body and the influences you are exposing it to than merely finding out how you brush and floss. The strength of your body's defenses and the environment you live in play a bigger role in controlling the threat of chronic inflammation and oxidative stress.

Dr. Ed Group, a chiropractor and healthcare practitioner in Texas, effectively summarized environmental influences on the body in one of his lectures. He lists some of the environmental influences your body is exposed to and the possible good and bad causes of degenerative disease and optimal health. He lists includes foods, beverages, bugs, stresses, EMFs, and toxins that should be avoided.[7] The good influences in the foods we eat and drink, the emotions we have and are exposed to, and possible healthy programs and solutions are also listed. Much of this information is available in more detail in his book, *The Green Body Cleanse.*

Table 4.2.   Ed Group's List

AIR	BAD: Lack of oxygen, mold and mildew, pet dander, building sickness syndrome, ozone and pollution, home AC filters, smoke and residue
	GOOD: Fresh air and filtered indoor air
FOOD	BAD: Meat, dairy, processed preservatives, digestive compaction, micro-waved, cooked, boxed, white flour, sugar, canned products
	GOOD: Fresh, raw vegetables and fruits, nuts, seeds, legumes, organic sources
WATER	BAD: Fluoride, chlorine, parasites, bacteria, heavy metals, reverse osmosis
	GOOD: Supercharged, distilled with organic apple cider vinegar, shower filter
BEVERAGES	BAD: Milk, alcohol, coffee, carbonated, bottled drinks
	GOOD: Herbal teas, soy milk, almond milk, rice milk, fresh vegetable juices
MICROBES	BAD: Viruses, bacteria, parasites, fungus, mycoplasms, yeast
	GOOD: Probiotics
PHYSICAL/EMOTIONAL STRESS	BAD: Fear, anger, depression, anxiety, jealousy, resentment
	GOOD: Hope, excitement, motivation, happiness, love, joy, relaxation
EMR/ME	BAD: Computers, cellular phones, big-screen TVs, digital clocks
	GOOD: Pen and paper, landline phones, analogue clocks, sundial
HEAVY METALS	BAD: Mercury, cadmium, aluminum, copper
	GOOD: None

This list is not comprehensive but it is a good start to understanding how the environment you live in must be taken into account and adjusted to if you are to obtain and maintain good health and vitality. Your health as a host is more important than the bad bugs and any other little physical influences. Forgiveness, love, and peace are far more important than the toothpaste, floss, or toothbrush you use. Focus on keeping the body in a higher, faster energy frequency because when you do this the bad bugs cannot invade as easily or survive.

KIRLIAN PHOTOGRAPHY

One of the ways we can actually see the energy of things around us and in our own bodies is called Kirlian photography. This technique records an image of the energy field around all living things.

You can see this energy field in and around plants, animals, and our own bodies. Healthy living things give off more positive energy than diseased

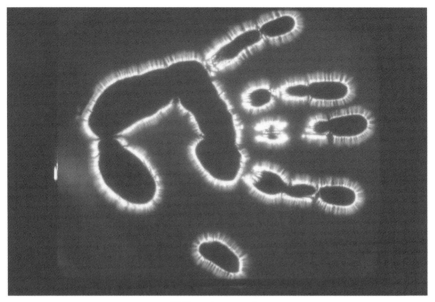

Kirlian photography
iStock.com/Absilom

or unhealthy tissues. This shows that we are more than flesh and blood. We have an energy field inside us as well as one that radiates to others and the world. Kirlian photography and other machines can now actually document the energy patterns coming from our bodies.

These photos of nature, the human body, and plants show the positive and negative energy flowing from the objects to the rest of the world. The energy that flows from you also flows outward and affects others and the rest of the world around you.

Some people have a gift to see energy fields of the body. The energy patterns of the body, flow out of different parts of the body in ever changing colors and patterns. These practitioners can see these patterns, their flow and colors, and also disturbances, changes, and problems in the energy systems that indicate health and disease.

EXPLORING CHAKRAS

Some practitioners have taken a slightly different view of the body and developed a system of energy patterns that influences us and radiates out to influence others. These are your chakras, which are energy patterns that radiate out of different levels of your body. They are constantly changing and

Chakras

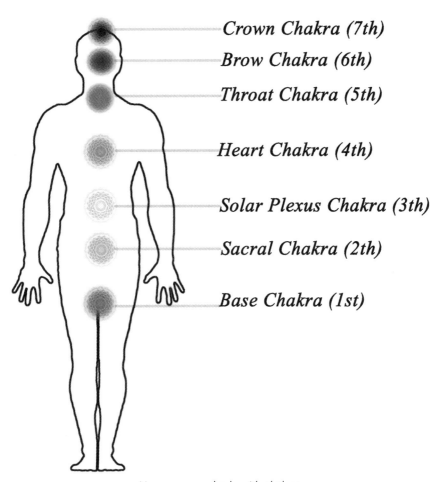

Crown Chakra (7th)

Brow Chakra (6th)

Throat Chakra (5th)

Heart Chakra (4th)

Solar Plexus Chakra (3th)

Sacral Chakra (2th)

Base Chakra (1st)

Human energy body with chakras
iStock.com/vaeenma

moving. They can change when you are unbalanced and diseased and move smoothly and bright if you are balanced and healthy.

I know some individuals who can detect, photograph, and even see these energy patterns. They can work with a person to get the chakras to brighten and move more smoothly. This work demonstrates the amazing way we were made and how we interact with the world around us.

MERIDIAN SYSTEMS

On a more intricate and defined level, Chinese and Far Eastern medical doctors have developed a vast system to describe the internal body's energy channels. These energy channels or meridians can be affected by the outside world and control the balance of energy—or chi—of the body. Acupuncture, acupressure, herbs, and healing touch are all used to bring these meridians back into balance and wholeness.

These meridians begin at the feet, go up the back, through the teeth, and back down the front of the body. Your teeth are all related to specific meridians. Blockage or disease in the teeth and gums can affect the energy and health of different parts of your body. For example, pockets of infection, heavy metals, poisons, implants, root canaled teeth, or cancer in the jaw can negatively affect the energy flow through your body. Remember in chapter 2, the chart showing how specific teeth are related to meridians.

When metal implants, root canaled teeth, or infections block a meridian, the rest of the organs, tissues, and systems on that meridian are also negatively affected. Clearing out the affected area can help restore balance and good health.

These meridians can be disturbed by dental infection and dental work.

Emotional trauma and negative emotions of fear, hatred, and a lack of forgiveness also can negatively affect these channels or meridians.

For most people, much of this might be a new experience, as it includes energy flow patterns and meridian systems that explain the physical and emotional balance of disturbance in a person. Once again, more information is available in the Resources section.

A new field in medicine and dentistry involves looking at, measuring, and treating the energy frequencies of the body. EAV machines detect and change the frequencies of the body to achieve balance. Treatments can be chosen that bring the physical and emotional body back into optimal health and vitality. Look to the future for practitioners to treat disease and imbalances with frequencies and energy medicine instead of drugs and poisons.

SOLUTIONS

So how can you and your holistic dentist use this information about your body and the world around you to stay balanced and healthy? Begin by focusing on the positive, faster, higher frequency things in your life. Don't obsess about every little unimportant thing.

I have patients who obsesses about each and every ingredient in natural toothpastes and miniscule contaminates in complex, healthy dental resins.

This fear is more damaging than any of the items they are so wary of and the anxiety is damaging their body more than any of the ingredients.

We obviously need clean, natural food, water, and air. Good filters can help a lot, such as quality HEPA filters for the air you breathe at work and in your home. Buy a good filter for the water you drink and use to cook your food. Eat fresh, raw fruits, vegetables, nuts, and seeds. Drink plenty of clean, filtered water, herbal tea, and fruit and vegetable juices. Use probiotics (or raw dairy and meats), natural supplements, and avoid electromotive forces (EMFs) with EMF pollution protectors, or limit all the EMFs you are exposed to, especially by your computer, cell phone, and TV.

Have the toxic metals in your teeth safely removed and replaced with non-toxic materials and then chelate your body of all the metals that have gotten into your liver, kidneys, brain, and central nervous system.

Find a good alternative medical M.D., holistic clinic, or life coach who can provide advice and testing, if needed.

Avoid negative environments, negative people, and negative feelings and spend more time in higher, faster energy places, with more positive people, and loving thoughts and feelings.

Find balance in your life between work, sleep, and play.

Most of us are caught up in work and school or a steady stream of activities and never find time to get adequate sleep or play. Our bodies work best with some down time. During sleep our bodies heal and repair and welcome spiritual things that we will get into later in this book. When it comes to play, choose fun activities because you like them and because they don't take a lot of mental thought, which is useful for grounding and real relaxation of the mind and spirit. This grounding does not have to be limited to sports or outdoor activities. Try walking with your bare feet in the sand or grass, swimming or wading in the water or walking in the forest or through desert trails. When we are grounding we are releasing negative energy from our bodies and gaining a balance or healthy energy from the world.

There is a growing amount of dental and medical research being done with quantum energy and physics. In the near future, bacteria, tissue, and the immune system will be diagnosed and treated with energy and frequency levels instead of chemicals, surgery, and radiation. EAV diagnostic machines, ion magnetic treatments for the body's own energy, low level lasers, and other health therapies will be used to obtain optimal health and vitality—with beautiful smiles as a bonus.

Look for dental and health practitioners in your area that are on the leading edge of these quickly evolving therapies and techniques that help balance your body and stay healthy for a lifetime.

A FINAL THOUGHT ON DOWNWARD CAUSATION

We were all taught in high school science class to look inward for the cause of why things happen. In the study of material science, this is called *upward causation* since the cause rises upward from the base level of the elementary particles, from atoms to molecules to bulkier matter, including living cells and the brain.[8]

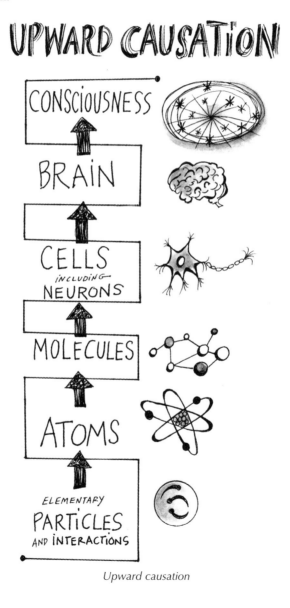

Upward causation

DOWNWARD CAUSATION

Downward causation

This theory is fine, except that according to quantum physics, objects represent waves of possibility and all that material interactions can do is change one possibility into another but never into any type of actuality we can experience. This is a scientific paradox of dualism, which asks us to keep an open mind to a changing universe.

To change possibility into actuality, a new source of causation is needed, which we can call *downward causation*. When we realize that consciousness is the anchor of all existence and material objects are possibilities of consciousness, then we also recognize the nature of downward causation. It consists of choosing one facet of a multifaceted object from a wave of possibility that becomes manifested as actuality.[9]

In our real world, it is not particles, atoms, and elements that create and change the world. It is our choosing. Cause comes from the top. Our atoms, DNA, or chemical reactions do not ultimately control us. We are controlled, changed, and transformed by our intentional choices. We are not automatic subjects to our DNA or "inherited" diseases in our families. We can co-create our own health and consciously choose balance and health over illness and disease. Transformation starts above and comes down through our choices, not up from our cells, DNA, and family history.

In the new quantum physics model, we can co-create possibility and actuality by downward causation. Prayers, intention, and free will choices create a shift in subtle matter, which can be mobilized into the real world. This can have wide ranging applications in the subject of health and healing. We can transform ourselves and help others do the same. Personal transformation through loving choices can trigger change in the entire world.

"So here we are, quantum activists, with the audacity of hope that we can change our worldview, change ourselves, and change the world," said the great anthropologist, Margaret Mead. "Never doubt that a small group of dedicated people can change the world. It is the only thing that ever has."

Each of us can make a difference.

Part II

OUR EMOTIONAL BODY

Now that we have established the essential connection between our teeth and gums and physical body, let's focus on our emotional body and how it affects our dental status and overall well-being. We know that effective dental care includes a diverse collection of genuine holistic treatment. As we begin to better understand how our body works we can also see the influence of our emotional lives on our overall health, and how taking care of that plays a vital role in an integrative program of dentistry.

Consider, for example, your physical body, something we can see, feel, touch, and smell. But isn't there more to being human than the body we occupy? We are more than a collection of cells and tissue. When it comes to interacting with others and with our environment, our *emotional* body—the one we can't see, feel, touch, or smell—is an equal partner and has great influence on the health of our physical body, including our teeth and gums.

In fact, significant scientific research shows how emotions can cause all kinds of illness—both acute and chronic. Some of these studies explain how emotional issues, such as stress, love, fear, lack of forgiveness, and pride, affect our daily health and can slowly but surely alter our physical body, including our hormones, immune system, and GI system, in positive and negative ways.

Part II offers practical actions you can take to reach optimal health and vitality in your life. These include creating a balance of work, play, sleep, forgiveness, and peace, leading to a discovery of how love can heal you, your loved ones, and the entire world.

5

Stress Busters: A Roadmap to Inner Peace

Most traditional doctors deal solely with the physical body. These practitioners break the body down into individual parts, learn how they work, and manipulate them to get you "well" through the use of drugs, surgery, and other techniques.

Complementary, functional doctors reach beyond a paradigm of physical parts and treat the body as a complex whole. Holistic research supports this approach, as it continues to show the beneficial, powerful healing effects of treating emotional body modalities along with, or sometimes in place of, traditional physical care. They are finding that healing can occur through love, compassion, laughter, and many other positive emotions. Some of these treatments account for up to 75 percent of the healing properties in a patient's treatment and recovery. Studies in psycho-immunology indicate that a positive mental attitude and the hope or expectation of healing can be powerful and even more effective than conventional medicines.[1] The energy of herbs and plants can also be harnessed to help handle the emotional body in a healthy way.

This chapter examines some of the root causes of stress in the environment and includes several positive solutions, including specific products and practices to reboot your emotional habits and set you on a better course. When patients learn to choose love over fear, peace over conflict, and victory over victimizing, they have healthier immune systems, less chronic inflammation, and better health.

Let's begin by exploring stress—what it is, how it works, and how it affects your teeth and gums.

THE ELEPHANT IN EVERY ROOM

Stress is the biggest trigger I see that influences the balance of the entire body. Negative stress influences five main areas of your dental health, all related to chronic inflammation and oxidative stress. They include tooth loss from depression and anxiety, psycho-immunological balance, teeth grinding, jaw problems, temporomandibular joint disorder (TMJD), energy indents, and a victim mentality.

These conditions can negatively influence the health of your teeth and gums, mainly through compromising the immune system, causing chronic inflammation, and upsetting your oxidative stress balance. The importance of oxidative stress cannot be overstated. It is the catalyst for a long cascade of health issues that ultimately wages war on the body's balance and leads to disease.

How you deal with stress can make all the difference in the world. Patients that can let it slide away like water on the back of a duck maintain healthier immune systems, experience less inflammation, and have fewer bouts with disease. They are able to adapt to change, don't allow daily stressors to mount up, and sometimes use natural plants and herbs to assist in their challenges with stress.

Prime One is an extraordinary product for maintaining overall health! It has been formulated with a scientific blend of rare plants called adaptogens. Adaptogen research began with famed Russian scientist, Dr. Israel Brekhman. After conducting approximately 1,200 studies on more than 1,000 plants, Brekhman isolated an adaptogen formula consisting of the strongest, most effective blend of adaptogens in the world.[2]

His formula is an exclusive ingredient in Prime One, which can help you achieve more energy, better sleep, and improved focus while reducing tension and anxiety. I include this product every day in my morning smoothie to keep my body in good balance and support my immune system. It gives me energy to work productively without fatigue, increases my capacity to focus, provides me with antioxidants, and balances my body to avoid getting sick. Prime One is one of the easiest ways to help your body cope with stress, and that includes your teeth and gums.

ORAL STRESS

Nowadays, as the world speeds up and our environment becomes less healthy, we are seeing more and more grinding and destruction of teeth and jaws and an increase in headaches. Many of my young patients have flat, worn down teeth from a grinding habit. Some adults I see have ground their teeth all the way to the gum line. The stress of difficulties in our finances, health, and relationships can influence the health of your teeth, immune system, and overall health. As we will see later, they can even be a factor in our spiritual life. These symptoms should remind us that the body must be treated holistically in order to establish and maintain optimal health and vitality.

How often have you found yourself clenching your teeth when you get mad or frustrated? How often do you clench you teeth when you simply remember a past event or person that has hurt you whom you have not really forgiven?

These emotions can trigger physical changes in the body, such as chronic inflammation, decreased immune system effectiveness, worn or flat teeth and cracked fillings, or headaches and migraines. Your emotional body, that is the stress you feel and carry inside you, can trigger any of these physical symptoms.

On the flip side, emotions of love and joy do not have these negative effects. Instead, they can have wondrous, positive effects on the body. Love and forgiveness can literally be healing, and we will explore how they work later in this section of the book.

THE BIG FIVE

Among the many factors that influence dental health, there are five in particular that I would like to explain, as they are the main disruptors to our well-being and the causes of many negative health issues.

1. Tooth Loss and Depression/Anxiety

In 2014, Constance Wiener, PhD, from West Virginia University, presented a report to the American Association for Dental Research , entitled "Association of tooth loss and depression and anxiety." She reported that although cavities and gum disease are the result of complex, chronic conditions, several bio-psycho-social factors are also involved.[3]

Some individuals in the study reported that dental anxiety played a role in their avoidance of dental care, while others suffering from depression revealed that they were negligent when it came to self-care. The study found a significant correlation between tooth loss and depression, anxiety, or a combination of both. Patients with depression and/or anxiety lost more teeth than the rest of the population in the study.

A patient that does not care about themselves or their dental hygiene will get cavities and/or gum disease and lose teeth. It does not matter if they have the best toothpaste with all the right ingredients, because if they don't care enough to pick it up and use it they will suffer the consequences. Without a genuine concern for their own health, they will not make an appointment to go to the dentist for regular check-ups or cleanings. These are prime examples of how negative emotions can affect the health of our teeth and gums.

When we consider everything we know about keeping our teeth and gums healthy forever, why do some people keep themselves from making them habitual? There is no physical barrier, no chemical product missing, or any biological reasons for doing so. The only missing thing keeping these people from achieving optimal health is the motivation to use the tools available to them. This is one example of how a lack of motivated self-care can influence one's health.

2. Psychoimmunological Factors

The second example of how the emotional body affects the teeth and gums comes from observing how your negative emotions can directly affect your body's immune system, nervous system, and balance. Since this is a large and complex field of research, we will only cover some of the basics here.

Psychoimmunology studies how your emotions affect changes in your physical body. For example, we know how the body is affected by positive stress, such as love, gratitude, and compassion. Significant research shows that a happy, joyful, thoughtful attitude can significantly affect healing outcomes. The heart beats faster, immune system cells form and speed up their function, and more oxygen flows to the cells, which function more efficiently and freely.

A new field of study documents how laughter and love heal and how a full range of positive emotions can change your cells, tissues, and organs. These changes are not triggered by chemicals or from biological tendencies. Instead, it is your emotional body that creates these effects—the magic of mind over matter, where your emotions can effect changes in your health and disease, which research currently being done is showing more and more.[4]

Conversely, negative emotions of yours or others around you can negatively affect your body and immune system. It is your immune system that fights off the bacteria that cause cavities and gum disease. The white blood cells that fight off these bad bugs can be turned on or off.

As we have seen through our look at energy levels in previous chapters, the low, slow energy of negative emotions can affect the whole body. Negative emotions, such as guilt, shame, and fear, are associated with low, slow, energy frequencies. If we stay in this state or around others who are in these states, we will negatively affect all the physical cells, tissues, and organs of our body.

The negative energy levels of all those around you can affect your body's health or disease. Living in an environment of anger, hate, or fear can affect your body. Living in a state of turmoil, pride, guilt, or greed will negatively affect you and your health.

3. Jaw Problems (TMJD)

One of the largest areas of the mouth affected by your emotions can be easily observed in those who are in the habit of grinding their teeth. Most of the patients I see have a loss of tooth height caused by this condition. If this grinding continues unchecked, problems will also arise in the jaw that supports these teeth.

Nowadays, most dentists deal with this condition by putting a piece of plastic in your mouth and letting you grind on the plastic. This protects your teeth as long as you wear the bite guard consistently. In some cases, we see patients that are so depressed that they may lack the motivation to wear the appliance.

This bite guard approach to a grinding habit does not address *why* a patient is grinding. Having a dentist treat the symptom without treating the cause is not ultimately helpful, either. Most people do not grind their teeth because they have a deficiency of plastic in their mouths.

This bite guard approach is another example of dentists trying to solve a symptom without looking at the whole person. They do not consider seeking to find the imbalance in the person's entire system that is causing the grinding. A calm, peaceful, balanced person does not grind his or her teeth. The cause of the problem may be outside the field of the physical body and more in the emotional and/or spiritual realm.

Most local dentists do not treat the whole body. Therefore, the causes continue and most likely worsen, leading to further destruction of the teeth and jaw joint.

There are some dentists beginning to look outside of the teeth for balance with a more holistic approach to the bite. These are neuromuscular (NM) dentists. They consider the balance of the teeth, gums, muscles, and skeletal structure when evaluating patients. By looking beyond the teeth and frequently working closely with chiropractors and other healthcare practitioners, they aim to balance the whole system through a more holistic and comprehensive perspective.

If you want a more holistic way to look at the physical body's influence when it comes to treating grinding and TMJD issues, a NM dentist would be a good place to start. Most dentists don't receive this training in traditional dental schools. There are places that train and certify dentists in this more comprehensive view of the teeth and jaw at the Las Vegas Institute (LVI), which teaches dentists to look beyond the teeth and jaw and consider the effects of the muscles, joints, and skeletal system for answers to a patient's imbalances.[5]

If you want to go even further beyond the physical body and look for other causes, you will need to search for practitioners that also address the emotional and spiritual body. We will address some of these concerns later in the book.

4. Indents

The fourth area of emotional imbalance is probably new to most readers and will take some explaining in order to describe the relationship to your teeth and gums. This is the effect of indents.

Over the course of my long career in dentistry I have often seen what I call "dental shoppers." They compare one dentist's fees for a filling, X-ray, or cleaning with another dentist's prices. This coupon shopper mentality treats healthcare as a financial commodity dictated merely by price and essentially ignores its substance. Most of my colleagues have seen the same thing and some of us do it, too, when it comes to other types of medical care.

It is an interesting habit, and most people that do it think they are smart in comparing different dentists by the cost of their product or service. This is a common misconception of the real world and we see it all the time.

The reality is, every dentist is different, just like any individual. For example, the toothpaste I sell in my practice is different than the same identical brand of toothpaste a patient can buy from some other dentist. The full porcelain crowns and cement I use is not the same as another dentist's full porcelain crowns and cement. The cleaning service my hygienists perform is not identical to the dentist down the street.

This is not because I am more special than another dentist. But I am different, and the services we provide are different because they emanate from a different energy, which ultimately affects your health and balance. When you compare what you consider to be identical services from two different dentists it often becomes a matter of comparing apples and oranges. Let me explain the difference.

Everything in the universe is energy. All matter has an energy level that can be measured. Everyone is affecting this energy with his or her own energy, or *indent*.[6]

This indent is like an energy label or address imprinted on everything you touch or influence. Everything that comes in contact with you or the area you are affecting has a positive or negative effect. If you are a negative influence, you put a negative indent on everything you come in contact with or influence.[7]

The orange you buy at the grocery store began as a seed planted by a farmer and his or her indent was put on that seed. A worker harvested the orange tree and he or she put his or her indent on that orange. The processor who washed, packed, or labeled the orange put their indent on the orange, too. The shipper, truck driver, packer, shelver, merchant, and cashier all put their own indents on that orange. The same orange from the same store may be totally different in energy from one in another store just down the block. They are not exactly the same product and have been indented in different ways.

When it comes to medical services provided, the differences can be even greater, especially when it comes to negative and positive influences between a patient and doctor. In this case, both parties play an equal role in how healthcare happens.

I try to buy products from companies with a positive influence, such as organic products that are not influenced by negative energy chemicals and toxins. I use non-toxic dental supplies and materials because some companies provide products with chemicals and toxins that have a slower, lower energy and may cause health problems for my patients. As a priest, I bless all the products and materials we use and sell so they have a positive energy influence on my patients.

The toothpaste I sell has been blessed and cleared of negative indents so they carry only positive energy to my patients. Every day at my office, I privately pray for the health of my patients and their families. I work in an office that is regularly blessed, consecrated, and protected from negative indents and spiritual influences, some of which we will discuss later.

Therefore, the services and products I provide are not comparable to the dentist down the street or at a lower cost clinic. People that compare them by price do not yet know they are comparing two different products or services. That's because prayer and intention changes the physical universe. Our emotional and spiritual health directly influences our physical body and the health of our teeth and gums.

5. Victimization

The fifth area of stress and illness in your body comes from your own internal self. We have seen the way love and gratitude affect water and the physical world. Now we will see how fear and stress can negatively affect your health and internal balance.

Let's look at an example from my dental office I see repeatedly among my patients—one that is becoming more and more prevalent in America, in general. That is people acting as a victim and blaming others and the situation for the wrongs they experience in life. Patients are caught up in blaming every one and every thing outside of themselves for the problems and conditions of their life. They are playing the victim.[8]

Let's look at one example through the story of Pat, who first came to my office for her initial examination appointment, which requires plenty of time to examine, evaluate, listen, explain answers to questions, and offer possible solutions to problems. But with patients like Pat, the standard one and a half hours can be too short.

The first indication of playing the victim appeared through her health questionnaire, filled out with full descriptions of every disease and condition in small print, filling all the space on the sides of the form and every margin, with full paragraphs explaining her troubling dental experiences and why they were not her fault. She told how the teeth were good at first and how her previous dentists and hygienists had ruined her teeth and gums. Similar blaming continued over and over with every new dentist she mentioned with an almost identical storyline.

The explanations blame everyone else but herself for the botched work and bad advice. She blamed relatives and friends for their bad advice, blamed bad toothpaste, chemicals in foods and drinks, a financial situation she has been forced into, and finally, Pat blames God for giving her all this to handle.

During the first part of an examination, before I start looking at anyone's teeth, I ask if there is anything bothering the patient or something he or she wants to make sure we address during the visit. Little did I know what this question would trigger in Pat, who used up most of the examination appointment telling her story.

Pat gave me a list of all the people, circumstances, and conditions that have caused her problems. She listed everything outside of her body that has been controlling her life and how she had no choice to make changes and was powerless to make things better. She described herself by her past hurts, family, feelings, situation, and circumstances. She was fixed in the victim role, frozen in fear, and unless she made a choice to change she would continue to be the victim for her entire life.

Fear is the opposite of love. Fear freezes people into the role of an inactive victim. As we saw before, the effect of love on water changes its environment. The same thing can happen with fear, which can change the whole body—and not for the better. Fear suppresses the immune system, tissue and organ function, and brings about disease.[9]

Fear, anxiety, guilt, and blame all negatively affect the water and cells of the body. Water is used in almost every chemical reaction in the body. Water is involved in everything your body does, every hormone, the energy your cells make, the repair and rebuilding that your cells control, the cells that fight off invaders, such as cavity and gum disease bugs, and all of what you need to maintain a healthy balance in your body. Being in a constant state of victimization and fear compromises your body's ability to function at its optimal level.

Pat will find it difficult to obtain and maintain optimal health and vitality and peace in her life with a victim's outlook and identity. She will always blame others and situations for her cavities, gum disease, pains, and infections. Even if I perform perfect dentistry, she will blame something or someone for the rest of her problems and pain.

Her problem is not the right toothpaste or flossing habit. It's not a lack of fluoride in her diet. Her problem is not primarily physical. For her, the solution to her problems in life will come from choosing love over fear, removing stress for peace, and eventually leading to balance in her life.

FROM VICTIM TO VICTOR

I wrote a master's degree thesis about the transformation from victim to victor, called "Victorious Living Through Self-Government." To make a long thesis short, the road from victim to victor begins with a question: Who or what is in control of your life?

Many situations and circumstances happen in our life that we may not choose but we are in control of how they affect us. We need to stop blaming other people, situations, and God for the influence these things seem to have over us and take responsibility for our choices of love or fear.[10]

When I see someone playing the role of victim, trapped in a cycle of pain and disease, I try to remind them that the reason they are behaving poorly is that they have forgot how powerful they really are, how beautiful life is, and how much they are loved by our Heavenly Father.

We can freely receive our birthright as a child of God created by love, in love, and for love. Love is the main reason we are here. This is why Jesus said the man was correct in summarizing the whole of the Old Testament law in his words:

> Love the Lord your God with all your heart and with all your soul and with all your strength and with all your mind, and Love your neighbor as yourself. (Luke 10:27)

Our free will gives us an opportunity to establish our own vision or life purpose. We take up our cross, confront the suffering, pain, or obstacles in our lives and stay true to our vision and purpose of our life. We trust God or some other source of energy to give us the talents and gifts needed to transform ourselves into victors.[11]

The three building blocks of transformation from victim to victor are founded on hope, faith, and love—hope in a vision, faith that God will provide, and love for others and ourselves. These building blocks will transform your heart and character to make transformation possible.[12]

Simply knowing these three words or concepts will not transform you. *You must take action.*

Patients playing the victim will always find other external sources for their problems, guilt, and pain. They will only break that cycle by changing thoughts, which change their emotions, which ultimately change their behavior and lives. They do this by creating a vision of their purpose for being here, setting goals, and keeping promises, which can be seen in their loving actions and results.[13]

Your love must be put into practical *action*, evaluated, and modified as needed by a changing environment. You must focus on who is doing the doing, and then you must act.[14] Ultimately, your vision will only become actualized when it is accompanied by love.

6

Love and Wellness

What does love have to do with wellness, and in particular, your choice of toothpaste? It's simple, as we can see from our previous discussion, because when it comes to taking care of our health we need to combine smart choices in the products we use with a loving approach to self-care. Both play a vital role in the health of our teeth and gums, as well as our entire body.

Let's begin with toothpaste, as it's the one oral product everyone uses. There are many brands of toothpaste to choose from and marketing popular brands costs millions of dollars. Long ago, before Madison Avenue took over on a grand scale, people were introduced to tooth brushing by using tooth powders and elixirs. The industry exploded when major commercial brands came on the market offering special promotions and advertisements, and soon they dominated the field by capturing the allegiance of individual consumers *and* dental professionals.

When fluoride entered the scene, the number of toothpaste brands multiplied and everyone assumed that it was an essential and healthy ingredient. If you look closely, you will see that none of the popular toothpastes on the commercial market list love as an ingredient—but it is the most important!

Why? Let's begin with the concept of energy levels and self-love, both of which play vital roles in our short and long-term wellness. Our energy levels can be affected by many different elements. For example, essential oils affect our energy levels, which play a role in maintaining a healthy metabolism and immune system. Some of these oils are edible and contain high energy levels. We can also see these valuable elements in the form of effective ingredients in toothpaste that can kill bad bugs, leave good bugs alone, and create a higher energy in users.

True love and wellness also means removing fear from our approach to good health. That process includes becoming informed about harmful chemicals we can avoid ingesting or coming into contact with, as well as reducing stressors, which affect our glandular functions.

We must also consider the love and energy put into the manufacturing, distributing, and selling of any holistic dental products, as well as the compassionate teachings a dentist should share with his or her patients—all with the intent of guiding people to wellness. We must always remember that love and gratitude can heal and that you are a co-creator of your body's health.

Remember Dr. Hawkins's energy chart in chapter 4 showing the scale of positive to negative energy levels. The author of the list associates emotions to each level of consciousness, which demonstrates that the physical world is closely bound to the emotional world and each has a different energy level.[1]

Everything is energy. All the individual ingredients in your toothpaste have an energy level, be it high or low. High energy levels pull you up and are healing. Low energy levels pull you down and cause disease. The ingredients in your toothpaste combine these energy levels. They are chosen to do specific things and perform different functions, but they also have energy levels of their own.

I recommend toothpaste that cleans plaque and food from teeth. They do not need food. They can't digest it, and have no need for food. They should be kept clean. I also want toothpaste that kills or inhibits bad bacteria and leaves good bacteria alone. I would like toothpaste to deodorize chemical odors in the mouth and leave the breath clean and fresh. Most of all, I want toothpaste that does no harm to a person, not to his or her teeth, gums, and entire body.

Here is a list of edible essential oils commonly used in healthy toothpaste and their energy levels.[2] Those with high energy levels are best to use for healing.

Table 6.1. Graph of Energy Levels of Essential Oils

Purification oil	46 MHz
Valor oil	47 MHz
Melrose oil	48 MHz
Basil oil	52 MHz
Sacred Mountain oil	176 MHz
Exodus II	180 MHz
Helichrysum oil	181 MHz
Joy oil	188 MHz
Forgiveness oil	192 MHz
Rose oil	320 MHz

I recommend a specific type of tooth and gum toothpaste to many of my patients, made by the Dental Herb Company, which combines essential oils, herbs, and green tea extract, which has been shown in numerous studies to be very effective.

The Dental Herb Company has conducted a lot of research and testing to come up with the combination of ingredients for their product. Some of this research can be found on its website—DentalHerb.com.

You can also create your own toothpaste by using the ingredients listed here, which are products that have been researched and proven effective in creating healthy mouths.

MAKE YOUR OWN TOOTHPASTE

Use Baking soda as a base and add your favorite ingredients: Green Tea extract, Turmeric, Grapefruit extract, Elderberry, Chinese Star Anise Oil, Colloidal Silver, Coconut Oil, Sunflower Oil, Sesame Seed Oil, Gotu Kola, Neem Oil, Thieves Oil (Clove, Cinnamon, Lemon, Eucalyptus, Rosemarius), Echinacea Purpurea Bud, Echinacea Augustolflora, Peppermint, Spearmint, Ocotea, Thymol, Wintergreen, Red Thyme, Lavender, Tea Tree Oil, Oregano Oil, Stevia, Xylitol, or Sorbitol.

You will need to experiment to find the consistency and taste you prefer. These ingredients have a high energy level (the energy level of love), which are effective and this energy indent for what goes into optimally healthy toothpaste is what I am referring to when I talk about including love in your toothpaste.

It aligns with the familiar phrase, "It's the thought that counts."

That's because everything you touch, hold, feel, or manipulate contains a certain energy indent connected to you. Every time you come into contact with any person or thing you get the energy indent of that person or product. That also applies to toothpaste, as we must consider all the people involved in the conception, manufacturing, distribution, and sales of these products, so by the time you're squeezing some toothpaste onto your toothbrush there has been a long chain of people and energy associated with you and your choice of toothpaste. Their indent and the environment it has passed through contribute in some way to your overall health.

The love and energy that each and every one of these people put into the product affects you either positively or negatively. This is why you want a product from a company that cares about the product and you as the consumer. These tend to be companies that use clean, safe, organic, unprocessed ingredients, conceived, produced, and consumed with love. Those are the types of products I highly recommend.

HOW YOUR CHOICES AFFECT YOUR EMOTIONAL HEALTH

Our emotional balance in life is influenced by a lot of things. Negative stress can hit us from many different sources—abuse, hurt, hatred, lack of forgiveness, just to name a few. How you deal with these stressful situations is a choice.

There are no accidents in how we relate to life. We all have accidents and encounter stressful situations but how we respond to them is no accident. It is a choice. How you feel, how you describe those feelings, and how you respond to them is no accident. You choose. You can play the victim, as we discussed earlier, and blame your circumstances, other people, or the world for your situation, or you can be the victor and view those challenges as learning experiences, mere steps to success or situations to respond to in order to ultimately achieve your vision.[3]

Two different people may respond to the same situation in different ways. For example, imagine an anxious dad driving a typical family car down a long, empty, dirt road, on his way to a family event. He pulls up to a railroad track, with lights flashing and the barrier arm down over the driving lane. Car by car, the train passes them by. The dad, anxious to get to the family gathering on time, rants and rages about the seemingly endless parade of train cars and the colossal waste of time sitting on the road waiting for them to pass by. He grows more and more angry at the train engineer for blocking his way and wasting his time.

His son, sitting excitedly in the back seat, is lost in his own dreams as he watches the endless variety of train cars passing by. The boy envisions strange people and exotic animals in the cars, traveling from distant lands on their way to wild adventures at their destinations. The blast of the train's horn further excites him and the clickety-clack of the train's wheel on the track fills him with wonder, that someday he might be able to ride in those cars or maybe become the engineer or conductor and see the world first-hand.

Father and son are in the same car, seeing the same situation, but they have totally different views of reality and how they choose to respond to it.

You are faced with the same thing nearly every day in how you choose to respond to your circumstances, how unexpected change may trigger your internal thoughts, and even challenge your belief system and the meaning of these circumstances. The thoughts you have—positive and/or negative—and the tendency you have of being the victim or the victor, will trigger and influence your emotions. They can be positive and healing or negative and unhealthy, ultimately causing some type of illness or disease.

You are the co-creator of your body's health.

THE BIG CHOICE

Your emotional health and balance ultimately depends on making only one choice in life: love or fear. Many things can affect your health and balance but this choice is in your control. This is one of the most important decisions that influences your health and balance—*not* the physical world around you.

Choosing love affects your cells' membranes, which affect the DNA inside them, turning proteins and genes off and on that control every aspect of your body. There is a good book by Dean Shrock, PhD, called *Why Love Heals* that goes further into the way love can affect your health and balance.

"Our core essence or energy pattern is love," he says. "When we experience love, when we resonate with our core essence of love, our bodies and being naturally absorb and align with this resonant energy. Health and well-being are the natural consequence of this experience. This is how love heals."[4]

I totally agree. Love creates a great and vibrant shift in our body, our relationships, and our personal health. Everything around us has the potential to shift to a positive and loving place. Our physical health shifts every time we make a choice motivated by love to attain more natural and balanced health.

If we choose fear then fear freezes us. It stagnates our progress and keeps us imbalanced and sick. Fear happens when we buy into the idea of unworthiness, separation, and doubt, essentially forgetting who we are. In these moments, we forget we were created from light and love, that we are children of God and have a divinely inspired purpose to share love with others.

Fears and lower energy—in you and around you—affects the water and all matter of your body. When you opt for fear, you inevitably destroy the balance and function of every cell and every organ and system that you need for optimal health. This can tear down tissues, stop your own defenses, and even cause disease.

Fear contributes to heart disease, cancer, ulcers, hypotension, tooth loss, teeth grinding, and many other conditions, which have been shown to be associated with your mental attitude. In some ways, I see fear and a lack of forgiveness as a bigger factor in gum disease and oral health than the choice of toothpaste brand and flossing habits.

The constant fear and anxiety some of my patients demonstrate is a small example of how they are affecting their own health. Many of my patients are overly concerned about the food, water, dental, and health product ingredients they are exposed to. Many are health conscious and always on the lookout for individual ingredients in the environment that can negatively affect their health and the health of their families. But some of them take this diligence too far and the fear that they have is sometimes worse than any of the individual ingredients they are fixated on.

Some obsess over every tiny ingredient in everything they see. They will not use a good toothpaste, such as the Tooth & Gums toothpaste I mentioned, because it contains an ingredient they don't like, in this case, a concern that carrageen, derived from seaweed, is going to cause their body harm. They obsess about the colored dyes in foods, the types of xylitol sugar substitutes, and every other ingredient in health products. They are good examples of worrying about every small tree in their environment while missing the benefit of the entire forest in front of them.

Constant fear and anxiety caused by worrying about every tiny ingredient in everything we are exposed to inevitably brings down the energy of every one of our cells, tissues, and organ systems. This worry about a seaweed ingredient in toothpaste is misguided, especially when that same person loses their teeth to gum disease they end up getting from the many dangerous chemical by-products that bad bugs emit, destroying the immune system and its defenses. They worry about eating enough organic kale only to be exposed to the thallium poison that the kale plant pulls from the soil and concentrates in the plant.

As we have seen, our bodies are not made to withstand constant stress and anxiety. Overtaxing our adrenal glands and nervous system will cause them to eventually break down. Working overtime to avoid tiny items in our food and drink often ends up taxing our systems in unreasonable ways.

I recommend that we focus on the big picture and let God handle the small stuff. Your body was wonderfully made to handle the small stuff and it has a beautiful capacity to adapt to changing conditions.

This list includes the 10 biggest chemical toxins we should try to avoid: Lead, Methyl mercury, Polychlorinated Biphenyls (PCB), Arsenic, Toluene, Manganese, Fluoride, Chlorpyrifos and DDT (pesticides), Tetrachloroethylene, Polybrominated Diphenyl Ether (PBDEs).

David C. Bellinger, PhD, MSc, a professor of Neurology at Harvard Medical School and senior research associate in Neurology at Children's Hospital in Boston, recently presented this information at the 13th International Symposium of the Institute for Functional Medicine.[5]

Your body's defense, immune, and elimination systems and your glutathione/selenium ratio, along with your prayers and intention, can handle all the small stuff when they are in balance. In the next chapter, we will provide helpful ways to help you stay in balance and achieve and maintain optimal health and vitality.

FORGIVENESS

A significant factor in determining your emotional health is forgiveness, and for some, a certain lack of forgiveness. When we hold on to grudges we are destroying our own bodies. This accumulation of low energy holds back our immune system, destroys cells and tissues, and allows disease to ravage our bodies. Not forgiving others, ourselves, and situations are one of the big issues you need to focus on—not the small stuff.[6]

Years ago, I helped a blessed lady by the name of Blessed Tiffany, who had been given a gift of healing people physically, emotionally, and spiritually. I had the privilege of being a "catcher" at healing sessions she held in California, where she served as a conduit for the healing energy of love that God would flow down to people through her.

But there were two reasons that could cause this healing *not* to happen. They both involved the patient's free will choice. God will not get in the way of our free will choice. He always gives us the choice to choose love or fear.

If we choose fear and deny forgiveness God will not interfere with our choice. Over and over, I observed two obstacles people could not get over— not feeling worthy of love and an inability to forgive themselves for the past.

They were holding a former lack of forgiveness, which created a barrier to love and light. This became their obstacle to optimal health and vitality. They had forgotten who they were and why they were here. They were letting a lack of forgiveness stand in the way of loving relationships, as well as physical and emotional healing.

Once in a while the person would crack open the door of his or her heart just a little and choose love over fear. When this happened, they could receive the physical and emotional healing they needed.

What always struck me was the power we have to choose love or fear. As co-creators of our lives, we have the power to influence how our bodies function and the emotional choices we make are immense and vital to our wellness.

Forgiving yourself as a way to achieve balance and optimal health should also be accompanied by an open mind and heart toward forgiving others. We live in a community of people bound to each other by interactions of love and fear. When we choose love and forgiveness the energy around us shifts to a brighter, healthier energy. A positive "ripple effect" happens when we interact this way with others, which offers us an inner peace and confidence, leading to better health.

Scientists have measured the positive effect of the human heart and found its effect can be measured up to 50 miles away.[7] This distance was chosen because this is the limit of the instruments they were using, but it probably goes on significantly further to impact others in your circle and in some cases, throughout the entire world.

When we choose fear and fail to forgive we create a negative effect all around. By not forgiving others we are bound to the one who hurt or betrayed us, and the longer we refuse to forgive or release the debt to those who hurt us the more our lack of forgiveness hardens into bitterness. When we hold on to this emotion and judgment toward another person, we do our selves no favors. But when we choose to love others with conviction, our hearts become lighter, our burdens are fewer, and in turn, our minds, bodies, and spirits will be healthier.

Think about it. When we do not forgive someone for a past offense, who hurts more—the other person? I don't think so. They probably have forgotten the offense and have moved on. If you are still unforgiving, mad, angry, or hurting, then you are the only one holding on to fear and harming yourself. You are destroying the water, cells, organs, and tissues of your own body. Your failure to forgive is eating at you and your body while the other person is free of any obvious harm.

The lesson is to forgive others even when they don't ask for it in order for you to stay healthy. Forgiveness frees you from being bound to the negative feeling and consequences so you can move on. Make a conscious choice to love and forgive every one. Remember the beautiful water crystals of love and gratitude and the opposite crystals influenced by hate and anger. This is what we do to our own bodies when we choose love or fear.

The last area of forgiveness involves forgiving a situation.[8] This is a little harder to understand and will be clearer when we explore the spiritual body influences in the next section of the book.

It starts with acknowledging that we are all fellow humans that make mistakes.

Sometimes, we need to forgive someone for a mistake or bad decision because we all can get into places and situations that overwhelm us and if we don't have the tools to ward them off we can fall under their influence, which can ultimately affect our health.

Anyone connected to religion and faith in any way knows that we were created by love, for love, and to love. We can choose to create a positive ripple effect inspired by this approach or we can trigger a negative ripple of fear, hate, and blame.

Choose love because it is our true birthright. We are meant to live in a spirit of love, forgiveness, and gratitude.[9]

After all, it's God's LAW: *Love Always Wins.*[10]

7

The Balance of the Universe and Your Teeth

When it comes to wellness, what does balance look like? What are some of the ways to achieve it in a hectic world full of toxins and an insufficient emphasis on achieving and maintaining optimal health?

This chapter will address the big picture of these issues, as well as specific things we can do—beyond simply choosing love over fear—by taking small, daily steps to create and stay in balance—physically, emotionally, and spiritually.

The process begins by controlling our thoughts and beliefs, governing our actions, and showing love to others by keeping our promises. When we are truly committed to these principles, we can better fulfill our mission in life, whether it's painting, building, healing, teaching, being a loving parent, a listening friend, or all of the above.

Any mission depends on a lifelong fulfillment of love. We human beings possess the right gifts and talents to accomplish our loving purpose in life—our destiny, if you will—so it is up to each of us to identify it and share it with the world.

As individuals, and as a collective society, we are too often spiraling downward into an abyss of apathy and despair. Many people—even in your family or among your neighbors—have lost their unique vision and purpose. They have deviated from the original design and path we were created to follow. Many in this world hide behind walls of blaming others, events, and circumstances—resulting in a lack of peace, joy, and love in their lives.

Traditional religions tell us that God did not create an original plan of endless pain, apathy, and death. He created a wonderful, beautifully designed, and self-perpetuating world of glorious possibilities and choices. We have been designed to exist in a community of love. We have only to accept that we are special children of the universe and here to share love with one another.

Years ago, my Masters thesis illustrated the broken path society is choosing, and prescribed a way out of these bad choices. It provided questions to ponder about our own choices and purpose in life. It described the transformation people choose, as they move from being the victim—letting people, things, or past circumstances control their life, to having a victorious life—filled with promise, love, and intimate relationships.[1]

This process starts inside each of us.

What are you committed to do with your life?

What obstacles will you overcome, to satisfy that commitment?

What have you been sent here to do, to accomplish or achieve?

Each of us has been made to love, but how do we find our path to unique achievements?

How do we discover our own genuine commitments? How can we show love to others and ourselves? Love will always guide us in finding the answers and making these decisions. Every choice that we make for love moves us ahead on our journey and it then becomes brighter. That is also the moment we can find joy and produce it for others.

Your purpose is a lifelong fulfillment of love. It is more like a complex arrangement of music that an orchestra plays. It is all the loving things that you were meant to share with others and the world. It can be just being a good friend, compassionate listener, thoughtful advisor, loving parent, helpful worker, powerful motivator, or thoughtful teacher.

Although we have the gifts and talents to accomplish our purpose, how do we do this loving work without becoming overwhelmed?

We do it by balancing three important areas in our lives: work, play, and sleep.[2]

Our entire physical, emotional, and spiritual body is made for a purpose, which is why we are here on Earth. If we only work, we will wear out this physical and emotional body. Work needs to be balanced with time to play or relax, as well as time to sleep and rejuvenate. Later, we will introduce the spiritual influences of play and sleep, but for now let's focus on the many emotional and physical aspects.

While you are working and active during the day, your body and spirit are actively working, too. Your body needs balance with playtime, just by doing something simple, easy, and fun. Sometimes, it may be something repetitious without a lot of focus. This is when the spiritual body can rest and play. It does not need to stay active and alert. Playtime for the body can be things like gardening, walking the dogs, playing games, or any number of hobbies.

You are more than your physical body. You affect the entire universe by everything you choose to do. All of this applies to general wellness *and* your teeth!

PRACTICAL TOOLS TO KEEP BALANCED AND HEALTHY

Grounding

Life is busy and can get overwhelming at times. During our busy schedules, we must make some time to relax and unwind. After all, our bodies are made to periodically rest—not just through sleeping. The Sabbath, whether that's observed on a Saturday or Sunday, exists to help humans rest and find peace—at least once a week.

Besides the spiritual practice of giving thanks in an organized sense, the Sabbath was created to be a day of rest. The body needs to rest and recharge, as well as our emotions. One of the best ways to do this, outside of a religious sense, is through what we call *grounding*.

Do you remember how your body relaxes and finds peace when you are resting at the beach, walking on a mountain path, swimming in the ocean, listening to a singing bird, or watching a beautiful sunset?

Any of these moments allows your physical body to rest and your emotional body to recharge. For example, when you are swimming in the ocean, you are connected to all the life in the sea. Your negative energy is diluted in the water and you take in the positive life energy of all the fish in the sea. The whole experience of swimming in an open ocean, peaceful lake, or clear, clean river, can help you relax and release negative energy and bring you back into balance.

Nature, a quiet spot in your backyard, a warm bath, a quiet time on vacation, or a peaceful time with animals, can ground your body and mind.

Find time each week to stop working and doing all of your normally rushed activities, so that your mind and body can truly relax. Enjoy the creation you live in and recharge your emotional body in this beautiful world.

PETS AS DELEGATES

One of the ways you can stay in balance is to share your life with a pet. Pets are here to help us through life. They are soul partners or special delegates, here to share unconditional love with you, helping you through physical and emotional pain as partners with you in this life.

Do you remember the energy chart earlier in this book? Energy levels above 400 are healing. The energy level for a dog wagging its tail is 500. The same energy level can be found in a purring cat or singing bird. These are all healing experiences and they can help keep you balanced and healthy.

Some of us are meant to have a delegate or a few delegates to help us through our lives. Without them, we would not be whole or in balance, and would be lacking in the help we need to get through this life more easily.

This is why, when a delegate dies, some people have trouble moving on or feel like a big part of their life is missing. Because delegates share themselves with us so openly and completely, when they are not around or die we are soon missing a piece of ourselves.

They can come back when we get a new pet, and we can have many delegates. They are here to help us throughout our lives, keeping our perspective clear, accepting unconditional love, sharing in our lives, and staying in balance.

PLAY

Play is whatever gives you joy. Play includes things you can do without much thought or work. These can be as individual as the person. For some, it is walking in nature, rock climbing, or swimming. Play may involve activities that sometimes can be repetitive, such as a hobby or video games, watching TV, or reading a book.

These are times that you find peace and joy in doing whatever it is that feels right for you and don't take a lot of attention to perform. Playing with a pet, throwing around a ball, or watching your children on the playground, all calm your body and mind. Without play, your guardian angel and spirit guides never relax. They become overworked and you tend to feel overwhelmed. Take time to play and relax or your physical body will start to break down, which will end up forcing you to slow down and rest.

DIET AND NUTRITION

What, when, and how we choose to eat is another way to be at peace. Organic, natural foods, made with love, contain a higher energy, are healthier, and can keep you in balance. The more processed, refined, and artificial food you consume, the slower and lower your energy will become, and the more you will have to struggle to stay in balance. In fact, if your diet is too out of whack, you will simply not be able to establish peace in your body at all.

A home-cooked meal lovingly made by a caring friend or relative can positively support your physical and emotional health. The person making the food puts their energy and intention into the food when they prepare it. They are literally sharing part of themselves with you when they cook and prepare your food, and in return, you are sharing your energy with them when you eat the meal with gratitude.

When you cook the food you eat, you lower your energy and the energy of your water, cells, proteins, organs, and tissues. That's because cooked food, especially using processed ingredients, kills good bacteria and enzymes in the food, which are naturally there to help us digest. Sometimes, we unwittingly change the shape of proteins and enzymes when we cook incorrectly, so that our bodies no longer recognize the food and do not know how to digest it.

Heavily processed foods, full of sugar and flour, can be quick and easy to make, but are not the foods our bodies are made to eat. In addition to changing the microflora (good bugs) in our mouth—seen in previous chapters—the processing changes the balance of hormones in our bodies that control the function of our cells and organs.

Lower energy food pulls down our emotions and slows down our bodies. Highly processed food factories do not add loving kindness and positive energy to their foods, like a caring mother, relative, or friend will do. The foods you eat can and *do* affect your emotional and physical body, which influence your general balance and health.

POSITIVE THINKING

For many years, researchers have proven over and over that a positive mental outlook on life can have a rousing effect on the body and mind. For centuries, we have been reminded of this effect because it is so important.

Whole industries and companies have been created to teach the positive effect that optimism, positive thinking, and hope can have on the function of the body, its immune system, state of mind, and spiritual health—in other words, our whole life!

We have seen how love and gratitude affect the structure of water. Optimism and positive thinking affect not only the water in our bodies but every cell. A positive outlook and perpetual hope can have profound effects on all your cells, organs, and defense systems.

You have probably noticed the negative feeling when you walk into a room where people have just finished a big fight. The tension and heaviness can be felt in the air. Your body can sense the negative energy because it can *feel* it as a simple reaction to the negative energy in the room.[3]

On the other hand, let's flip the script to when you can sense a positive energy in a room when it is filled with positive people, with some even radiating enough loving energy that you can feel it affecting you with its positive intention.

This positive emotional choice, by you and the other people around you, of love, kindness, forgiveness, and gratitude, can affect your body, those around you, and the whole universe. That's because we can actually see energy flowing from our bodies.

PRAYER AND INTENTION

Beyond these largely physical methods to balance the body, we can also turn to prayer and positive intentions, two powerful tools to help rebalance and recharge the body. Prayer and giving thanks can change the water and the substance of the things and people around you. Pray over the food you eat, the drinks you enjoy, the medicine and products you use, your home, car, kids and spouses, hotel rooms, planes and trains you travel in, stores you visit—everything.

Pray over the toothpaste and mouth rinse you use. Pray that they do not have any negative effect on you and only a positive healthy effect on you and your family. Pray a prayer of protection and thanks for the people you care about, that they stay safe from any accident or problems.

I send a prayer of blessings over every store I enter, every building or business I enter, every hotel room I stay in, and every restaurant where I dine. I ask that the person, place or things be blessed and all negative influences be rinsed clean. If you are so inclined, you can do the same thing to everything you are exposed to, every loved one you encounter, everything you come into contact with. Your positive, loving, and healing energy can positively affect all those around you. How wonderful the world would be if everyone did this—in their own way—to find peace, emotional and physical healing, and balance, through loving prayer and positive intentions.

BLESSINGS

The last way of finding and sharing emotional peace and healing with those around you is through blessings, expressions of wishing happiness and prosperity to someone. It is wishing to send to others love, hope, good fortune, and joy.

One of the reasons we are here, living out our lives, is to love and serve others. One of the easiest ways we can help others is by wishing the best for them and offering them blessings. A simple thought or statement of blessing you send to others can have a positive effect on them and their lives.

You can bring positive, healing energy to yourself and other loved ones by blessing your homes, cars, business, and property. The use of holy water, blessing oils, and the presence of a special loving object in a home, can help heal and balance an area.

There are special blessings and prayers called *the Divine Decrees*. I mention them now because of the positive affects they can have on your emotional health and the health of others around you and the entire world.

Blessings can help create peaceful, loving homes and relationships. Blessings that a home receives from a priest or pastor can protect it for a period of time, land can be dedicated to holy ground, and people and places can be cleaned of negative indents and influences.

For those of you especially interested in this, there is much more to share about the power of blessings, but it will have to wait for my next book.

All of these things are ways to positively affect your emotional body and consequently your physical body, too. You and the entire world are affected by your choice of love or fear. This choice of love affects us, and others around us, and the subsequent energy flows out into the entire world.

Love and light start within each of us and can be a powerful influence on our balance, as well as the health and balance of others in our families and communities. This positive change can transform the entire world, and it all starts with individual choice.

Part III

OUR SPIRITUAL BODY

Many of you may wonder what our spiritual body has to do with our teeth or general health, and why I've chosen to include this topic in a book on holistic dentistry. Once again, *authentic* holistic treatment of any kind—for the teeth, brain, or liver—must also consider our emotional well-being, which we've surveyed in Part II, as well as our soul and spirit, and how it may influence the care of our teeth, gums, and overall health.

This is difficult terrain to explore, let alone explain, but probably not for the reasons you may think. As a man of science *and* a priest and chiropath (a God-centered healer), I have encountered miraculous healing experiences, explored the expanding limits of our knowledge of the universe through quantum physics, and opened my mind to the influence of the heart. In all of these instances, I have seen how choosing love affects our physical and emotional body.

Inside each of us, within our physical, emotional, and spiritual existence, an energy resides together inside our singular body, even if it doesn't always feel that way. For example, when these three elements are not operating in positive harmony with each other, we can become ill in any number of ways—acutely, for a limited time, or through some chronic condition, which may continue for years or a lifetime.

My philosophy is to always consider the physical, emotional, and spiritual aspects of any individual living being, with no real separation, as they are intimately intertwined. When I consider one aspect, I really end up treating all three together. This is the central point of any effective wellness concept and the anchor of a true holistic approach.

I believe that spiritual health affects everything we do in life, and in many cases its influences are the strongest and most important. This occurs through

133

individual free will, our deep connection with others, and for some this includes encountering spiritual entities and God. All these connections and choices greatly affect the balance and health of our body and those around us.

No matter what you may believe (or not) when it comes to a Higher Power, I think we can all agree that our state of mind and the condition of our deeper levels of existence play a pivotal role in our overall health. Keeping an open mind and paying attention to our spiritual heartbeat can help us develop a richer understanding and sensitivity to ourselves and the world we live in, which ultimately can help us achieve optimal vitality and health. And the key to all of that is love.

8

Love and Healing

What if you started playing a basketball game that you knew you were go-ing to win before you even began? You knew that even when your team was down 10 points and you missed a free throw, in the end your team would win the game. Would it make you feel different, even while playing hard and missing a few shots in a row—that your team would still win? Would you look at small setbacks and a missed shot differently?

These small setbacks may not bother you, knowing that they didn't matter in the end. You may play with more peace, have more fun, and not get so upset when small problems happen during the game. Others may look at you and wonder why the little things going wrong are not upsetting you. Some of the people watching may want the same peace, love, and balance that they see in you.

They haven't yet figured out the role of spirituality in your countenance, and how they can make such a big difference in your daily wellness. In this chapter, we will explore love, forgiveness, prayer, intention, and a connection to a higher source. This includes the ongoing need most of us have to forgive someone for making a mistake or a bad decision we make because of letting others influence or control a situation. We all run into moments and events that overwhelm us, and if we don't have the tools to ward them off we can fall under their influence.

Our society frowns on talking openly about politics, sex, or religion. I will introduce you to some of the ways your health is influenced by the universe outside of your physical and emotional body, and how choosing love and forgiveness can help us grow and thrive.

After all, love always wins.

WHAT IS *DIS*-EASE?

How do people become trapped in chronic illness? Beyond our genetic dispositions, might it also be a result of fear, anxiety, a loss of free will, and individual choice, or the ruthless pull of numerous addictions? When any of these afflictions become too strong, *dis*-ease will occur, and in many cases it will persist and even worsen without the type of intervention that spiritual healing can provide, which can vary, depending on one's inclination, curiosity, and/or religious leanings. It may transpire through a specific healer or by virtue of an individual's search for a deeper and stronger connection with their respective faith and the power and wonder of God's love, whether that is manifested through traditional means or by a simple abstract belief in energy forces beyond our scope of comprehension.

LOVE VERSUS FEAR

Every day around the world, people find healing without drugs, medicine, nutrition, or surgery. They do not rely on one's emotion or even being conscious when the miracle occurs. We could say this is the result of a mindset, declaring that we might simultaneously be realistic *and* expect miracles.

For some people, choosing love and light over fear and darkness can be the key to improving their health. Love and light are a free gift available to all of us, if we choose to embrace them and reap their benefits. Each of us has the capacity to make this shift in our life—from fear to love, and when we do so in a genuine way, it may even alter the chemistry of our body in surprising ways, leading to levels of healing we may not have thought were possible.

Some people are resistant to accepting the idea that our spiritual life can affect our physical and emotional well-being. One reason may be when that person is too intellectual, when his or her right side of the brain, which controls logic, has difficulty accepting spiritual healing. But those who decide to take a chance and venture outside their usual comfort zone—even when they do not fully understand the process—can discover a flow of healing and love previously unknown to them

This requires shutting off the analytical right side of the brain to overcome this obstacle. These people tune out for a moment, whether it comes through a religious rite or ceremony, listening to emotional music, or meditating. It requires letting go of the conscious emotions we normally experience and opening the door to new energies. I have seen these influences work time and time again, healing people of all sorts of conditions and illnesses. Even dental conditions can be healed this way.

THE CONCEPT OF FREE WILL

What allows one person to be healed and not another? I believe it is a matter of simple *free will choice*. Remember how the layers of the body were described earlier? The physical body inside is surrounded by an etheric body radiating outward. Think of this free will space as a bubble or impenetrable force field outside of your physical and etheric body, which creates a protective and powerful force field of spiritual energy and positive influence.

We can choose to be open to the possibility of healing, and when we do we forgive and accept love, allowing us to receive healing. The biggest obstacle to this is not choosing the right physical drug, medicine, or surgery. When we realize that we can choose love over fear, be gentle and forgive ourselves (and others) we then can allow ourselves to become worthy of genuine love, the ultimate gateway to healing.

When we choose fear, we put holes in our spiritual bubble of protection by allowing negative influences to affect our lives and those around us. For example, an addiction to sex, drugs, or damaging behavior can allow negative influences to pour into our lives. We can prevent this by choosing love over fear, bad habits, and addictions, by choosing to forgive ourselves and others, and even challenging situations. We can clear out negative influences and fill these holes with love and light.[1]

If you are interested or so inclined, there are simple prayers to rid yourself of these negative influences and simple loving habits to change, which can keep you on the path of making the right choices.

WATER AND LIFE

Negative influences are related to the physical world, which we can see in the world of quantum physics. These negative spiritual influences are the slow, low frequencies of despair, anger, and hate, which are destructive frequencies that can cause illness, hopelessness, depression, and death. These forces can tear down the world and destroy everything that is good and loving.

Take the simple example of water, which has fascinated scientists for years. This simple substance has amazing properties—exactly what we need to maintain life. Some scientists have taken simple water and changed it with physical, emotional, and spiritual influences. It's not hard to do and is a simple test.

Dr. Masaru Emoto came to the conclusion that human consciousness can alter the molecular structure of water, which is not hard to imagine when we remember that our bodies are made up of 75 percent water and the world around us can be influenced all the time by negative and positive energy.[2]

For the most part, you choose what you put in your body, who you love or fear, what you read or listen to, where you live, work, or play. All your choices affect you, your family, and friends, and ultimately the whole world.

FREE WILL BEFORE BIRTH

According to this belief, you are here on earth at this time and place for a purpose, with a chosen path to follow and something to accomplish in some aspect of your life. Those who ascribe to this concept, which includes religious people of multiple faiths all around the globe, believe that you choose the human body you were born into. You choose your mother and father and your family. You choose the gifts you have and the consequences of your body, the family, and time to be born. These are all the choices you made before you were born.[3]

We must remember that some things happen once we get here that we do not control. Accidents, other people's choices, sin, death, indents, and manipulations can all happen, but many of these are main choices you made and knew about before you accepted to come back to this present life.

Some of our choices are for our own good. Gifts you have and were born with are an example. If you choose to develop them they can be for the ultimate good—for you, your family, and the world.

Some of the choices we made are for the good of others and to learn from. Some of us choose weak bodies, bodies predisposed to health problems, emotional family problems, and spiritual battles.

Most of the illnesses, weaknesses, and health problems stem from our own choices. What we eat, how we exercise, how we rest, play, and sleep is all in our control.

HIGH AND LOW SPIRITUAL FREQUENCIES

As we have seen in previous chapters, everything is energy, from a very high level to one very low. We see the same thing in the spiritual universe. You may have heard of cursed objects or heard about someone putting a curse on something or someone. These use negative influences and negative energy and are connected to a physical object or person.

Evil people can hurt those who have holes in their free will. It is like a spiritual address on an envelope, which follows the envelope or object wherever it goes. The evil indent influences anything it comes into contact with. It can lower your energy enough to make you sick, have evil thoughts, and adversely affect your emotions.[4]

Some people are very sensitive to these indents. They are gifted enough to recognize them and help these people get rid of the evil indents, close free will spaces, and keep them closed.

Things can also have a good indent on them. Blessed objects, people, places, holy water, holy oil, churches, synagogues, monasteries, crucifixes, crosses, light, and love all can have a positive influence in your life. Fill your hearts and the universe with good intentions, loving objects, light and love, forgiveness, and gratitude.

FREE WILL PROTECTION

Choices before birth, indents after, and your own current free will choices are spiritual influences that can affect your health. All three of these choices make holes in your free will protection. Doctors can't help you heal from these bad indents or your choices. These are your choices and you can heal them, if this is your choice, if it is your purpose in life and your commission.

You may have noticed that I have not yet brought up religion. This is not a religious book, per se, but I would like to remind you that whatever your religious center may be, it is a powerful healing avenue for your health and can play a significant role when it comes to finding solutions for whatever health problems you may have.

But religious life can also be a negative influence. It can push people away, through hypocrisy or concepts constantly dealing with shame and guilt. This is a big topic for another day, if not another book.

Let's return to the concept that the world is a mysterious place and we cannot always understand it or even rely on science for explanations. That is where our inner *and* outer spiritual lives come into play, and where the process of real healing resides—somewhere in between the laboratory and our hearts and minds, and souls.

Our health depends on many factors, and it's in our best interest to take responsibility for everything we can control. But then again, if we have an open mind and heart, we can also be realistic and expect miracles.

YOUR SPIRITUAL TOOLKIT

Some patients have unexplainable, prolonged, or unusual health problems. Some seem overwhelmed by problems passed down through generations in their families. But even if one has balance in the three primary areas of his or her existence—physically, emotionally, and spiritually, he or she may still not be experiencing wholeness and perfect peace.

A person in this situation may require a *fourth* level of healing, one that addresses influences outside of us—negative drags on our finances, health, or relationships that could arise from a universe outside of ourselves.[5]

In that case, specific healing tools are needed, including prayers and blessings, so you and your family can be transformed into a more peaceful and happy place, and when coupled with the power of intention can calm storms, reduce conflict around the globe, and bring peace to places of strife.

These tools can change your health, too. When we send healing energy to the past, we can also transform that future and begin to heal the entire world. I've chosen to include reference to this fourth world simply because some of you may be interested to pursue this approach. If that is the case, you can find more information on my website or through many other sources available online or perhaps in your local community.

PROTECTING YOURSELF AT HOME AND IN BUSINESS

As you become brighter and choose love, this will create a ripple effect around you. Just as the circular effect that happens when you toss a pebble into water, your energy will also expand to the world around you, including your family, neighbors, friends, and community.

You may be overwhelmed by the darkness of the world. The news is full of hate, protests, rebellion, and war. Choose love and gratitude anyway.

There are a million acts of kindness and charity that happen all over the world at every moment. These rarely get the headlines, but play an important role in transforming the world for the better, and chances for this increase when each of us choose love over fear, gratitude over hate, forgiveness over revenge, and light over darkness.

Dr. Emoto's study of the transformation of water demonstrated among other things that love and gratitude can influence the physical world and create beautiful effects. They can also transform your body. This ripple effect will show in tangible benefits to your physical, emotional, and spiritual well-being, and this transformation also has the capacity to change the whole world.

Your home and businesses should be a place of peace, rest, and service. I have given you some of the ways to create a spiritual connection in your surroundings. These are things everyone can do to co-create a little bit of heaven on earth.

We are asked to have a clean and bright place especially where we live, where we may be unencumbered by anything that is not existing in an energy of love, that we may be in a place of brightness without manipulation or connected to things that are of a lower vibration.

As you know, love and light have a ripple effect. We are all connected. All the people in the world affect each other. Each and every place in your home, neighborhood, and city can be blessed and protected.

As we explored in chapter 4, the ripple effect and its power to transform the world is beginning to be understood by scientists. Those who study quantum physics are becoming more and more cognizant of the fact that all is connected and everything affects everything else. Although the quantum physics field is immense in scope and details and expanding all the time, some of what it offers supports the theories of how love and energy affect our health and the well-being of the world.[6]

We make changes in ourselves by choosing to change our mindset and co-create new thinking that manifests light and love.[7] This conscious choice manifests in the real world and changes our energy, life style, and health. When we change ourselves and our environment, the ripple effect starts to change the entire world.[8]

EVERYTHING IS CONNECTED

One of the most important concepts of quantum physics is that everything is connected. Everything is energy and affects everything else.[9]

When we hate, succumb to anger, become bitter and yell, protest, or fight, we are using a lower, slower energy that is unhealthy and weakens ourselves and all those around us, and eventually spreads out to affect people everywhere.

We can choose love, instead. We can opt to practice loving care for our body. We can choose forgivingness of ourselves, others, and the situation instead of choosing hate, anger, and revenge. We can choose to make a difference in people's lives and the environment and this can transform the entire world.[10]

At the center of this for each of us is our health—physical, emotional, and spiritual—and the spiritual "tools" we have at our disposal can be used to improve your health and transform your life, the lives of those around you, and the entire world.

ESTABLISHING A SPIRITUAL CONNECTION

We get busy with life, kids, sports, work, and all of the hectic living. As a result, we are susceptible to losing the peace, love, and connection to our spiritual selves that we are capable of experiencing. We can do this in lots of ways. Many of these tools will make your life happier, more peaceful, and less stressful, which all lead to better health.[11]

Create a Sacred Space

You can create a peaceful, quiet space in your home that you can go to and relax, focus on your faith, and reconnect to your inner spirit.

Arrange an inside "altar" in your house with objects that hold a special place in your heart, inspire you, and bring you happy memories, or just create a space for peace and love. An outside altar area could contain some special stones, driftwood, a statue, or waterfall. Hanging plants or flowers, herb plants, chimes, or a fishpond can also work. This is a special place to relax, unwind, find peace, rebalance, and connect with the love in your heart.

Meditation

Quiet times to just be with God and talk with Him can be powerful. By being still in your spirit you can listen to the still small voice of God in your life. Spend some time away from the constant noise of the TV, computer screen, or cell phone. Even 20 minutes of prayer and meditation can lower BP, ease migraines, calm colitis, and help cure a number of ailments.[12]

Taking a Break

Periods of fasting and rest can give you more balance and answers from God. Church sponsored retreats, self-planned sabbaticals, periodic days of fasting and prayer can give the physical body the rest and cleansing it sometimes needs to be working at optimal health and vitality.[13]

Church

Gathering yourself together with others in a center of worship, such as a church, synagogue, or mosque, can lead to a closer connection with God. They offer fellowship, support, and rest to their members and guests. Time spent in these settings can help resolve conflicts, give encouragement and praise, and lead to a closer communion with your Father.[14]

MAKING THE MOST OF YOUR SPIRITUAL TOOLKIT

This chapter has given you some of the tools to help you stay in spiritual balance. While we are spiritual beings having a physical experience, our

Loving, Heavenly Father longs to help His kids in all areas of their lives. He has given us ways to communicate with Him in prayer, opportunities to help change this world for the better with blessings, Holy water, divine decrees, and ways to stay connected through items, sacred places, and other people—always with the intent of sharing love. These are some of the tools we have available to us to compete in the basketball game we described as a metaphor at the beginning of this chapter.

Remember that love always wins and that you will always be on the right side if you choose love instead of fear, choose to be a light in the darkness, bless and forgive everyone, and stay in touch with your spiritual self.

This is the key to righteous living and optimal health.

Conclusion

Your Path to Optimal Health

Let us conclude our journey with a review of new trends in contemporary dental treatment, specifically how we are crossing the bridge from relying on the status quo to embracing the benefits of integrative and *authentic* holistic treatments.

Our holistic approach to wellness enables us to view health through a physical, emotional, and spiritual triad. This model reinforces the value of unconditional love, forgiveness, gratitude, balance, and the exciting potential of alternative medicine.

This also suggests a need for continuing education and integrative research that can move the needle in the direction of making the most of what holistic healthcare can offer—the opportunity to inspire individuals to focus on wellness and a healthier society, with an optimistic view of the future.

YOUR ACTION LIST

Dental

In order to maintain good teeth and gums, see a good holistic dentist regularly for cleanings and check-ups, avoid toxic poisons, use effective toothpaste, mouth rinse, Lolozs lollipops, Dentiva, and MI paste, as needed, eat a fresh organic diet, and try to maintain a healthy immune system.

Medical

In order to decrease inflammation and oxidative stress, eat foods based on your body type and see a holistic medical doctor regularly for advice.

Nutrition

In order to establish the best habits for you, find your body type, balance proteins, carbohydrates, and fats, stay in the Zone, cleanse regularly, and decrease your intake of sugar, gluten, and processed foods.

Stress

In order to lower your stress, choose to be a victor instead of the victim, decrease tendencies to be overly prideful and increase humility.

Love

In order to love others, you must first love yourself and the situations you are in, which will be easier when you forgive everything and everyone and find your purpose in life.

Balance

In order to sustain a healthy life, find a balance of work, play, and sleep— about one-third each, which will help you stay grounded and find and maintain peace in your life.

Free Will

In order to own the blessings of free will and stay in love and light, choose love over fear, cleanse your free will space regularly, and use prayer and intention on a daily basis.

Universal Responsibility

In order to bring yourself joy, find your purpose, fulfill your promises, have hope in your vision, faith in your unique gifts and unselfish love for everyone. Be an instrument of peace, love, and joy to all those around you.

World

In order to change the world locally and globally, seek higher and faster energy everywhere, and learn to balance and ground yourself.

God's Law

In order to live a blessed life for yourself and others, embrace the idea that love always wins, that prayer and thanksgiving are always there for you, and that life is a gift.

BALANCE IS THE KEY

Just as this book focuses on physical, emotional, and spiritual health, our main desire must be to achieve and maintain balance in each of these dimensions—through our own actions, with the advice of professional experts, and for those inclined, through prayer.

People in physical balance have certain qualities that they maintain. They eat and drink a responsible diet of fresh food that matches their body type, maintain healthy habits to keep their teeth and gums clean, and do the same for the rest of their body.

People in emotional balance are able to deal healthily with stress. They are humble, loving, and forgiving, and serve those around them. They work hard at what gives them joy, balance it with play to restore energy, and are at peace.

People in spiritual balance shine forth in their personalities like luminous beacons in a foggy night. They love without judging others, understand that the Divine Spark is within everyone, and see each person as a child of God.

When someone keeps all three of these systems healthy, they are not only taking responsibility for themselves and their immediate family. They are also caring for others in their community and for the environment as a whole. This is done through unconditional love, forgiveness, and gratitude. They know love!

What a wondrous life is potentially attainable for every human on the planet, and I hope this book can play a role in helping you open your heart to this idea.

I wish you peace and love. I pray for all of you daily, that you will come to forgive everything and everyone. I am here to help you in whatever way I can, but you have to make the choice to embrace these possibilities.

Choose love, because love always wins.

Blessings,

Rev. Dr. Stephen A. Lawrence

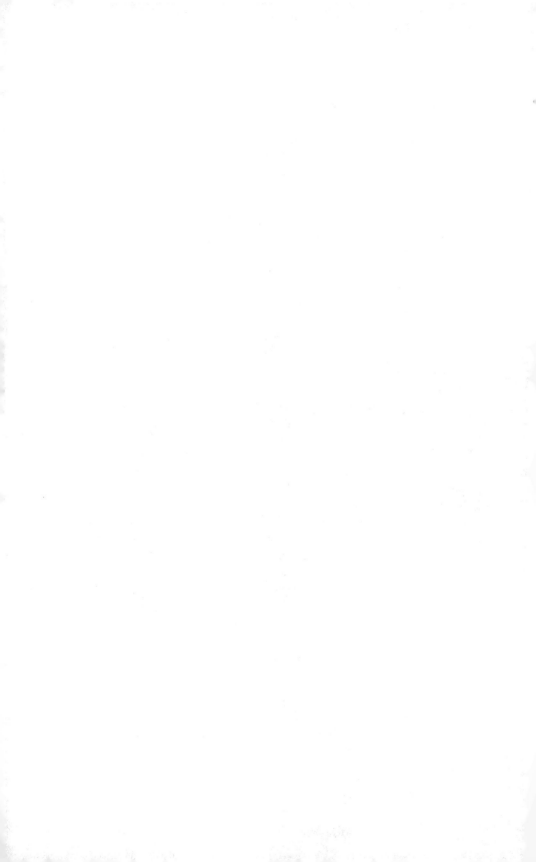

Notes

INTRODUCTION. HOLISTIC DENTISTRY: A COMPREHENSIVE APPROACH TO HEALTH AND WELLNESS

1. John P. A. Ioannidis, August 2005, "Why Most Published Findings Are False," *Plos Medicine,* 1–10. plosmedicine.org/article/info:doi/10.1371/journal.pmed .0020124.

CHAPTER 1. DENTAL HEALTHCARE 101

1. Christina J. Adler et al., "Sequencing Ancient Calcified Dental Plaque Shows Changes in Oral Microbiota with Dietary Shifts of the Neolithic and Industrial Revolutions," *Nature Genetic,* 2013 (45), pp. 450–55. DOI: 10.1038/ng.2536.

2. Weston Price, DDS, *Nutrition and Physical Degeneration*, 1997, 6th edition, Price-Pottenger Nutrition Foundation, La Mesa, CA, xv, xvi, 1, 300, 472, 474–75.

3. J. A. Aas, et al., "Defining the Normal Bacterial Flora of the Oral Cavity," *J Clin Microbiol,* 2005, Nov.; 43 (11): 5721–32.

4. A. L. Davey and A. H. Roger, "Multiple Types of the Bacterium Streptococcus Mutans in the Human Mouth and Their Intra-family Transmission," *Arch Oral Biol.* 1984; 29 (6): 453–60.

5. Juan Houte, "Role of Micro-organisms in the Caries Etiology," *J Dent Res*, 73 (3): 672–91, March 1994.

6. Ernest Newbrun, *Cariology*, 1989, Quintessence Publishing Company, Microflora chapter, 44–75.

7. J. W. Costerton and Philip S. Stewart, "Battling Biofilms," *Emerging Trends in Oral Care*, Scientific American, Inc., New York, NY, 2002, 6–12.

8. Pamela R. Overman, RDH, MS, "Biofilm: A New View of Plaque," *J Contemporary Dental Practice*, vol. 1, no. 3, Summer, 2000, 1–8.

9. D. Sambunjak et al., "Flossing for the Management of Periodontal Diseases and Dental Caries in Adults," *Cochrane Database Syst Rev*, 2011 (12): CDOO8829, Pub 2.

10. Maxwell Anderson, DDS, MS, Med, et al., "Modern Management of Dental Caries: The Cutting Edge Is Not the Dental Bur," *JADA*, June 1993, vol. 124, no. 6, 36–44.

11. Pamela R. Overman, RDH, MS, 2000, ibid., 1–8.

12. Pamela R. Overman, 2000, ibid., 1–8.

13. Ken Southward, DDS, FAGD, "The Systemic Theory of Dental Caries," *General Dentistry*, September/October 2011, vol. 59, no. 5, 367–73.

14. Ralph Steinmen, DDS, MS, and John Leonora, PhD, "Dentinal Fluid Transport," Loma Linda University Press, 2004.

15. Bill Landers, "How Fast Do Bacteria in Your Mouth Grow?" Oratalk, Fall 2006, 3.

16. A. Tadinada et al., "The Evolution of a Tooth Brush: From Antiquity to Present—A Mini Review," *J of Dental Health, Oral Disorders & Therapy,* 2015, 2 (4) 00055DOI: 10.15406/jdhodt 2015.0200055.

17. Brian Novy, DDS, CEA Dental Convention lecture, *The Cutting Edge of Caries Management*, November 2007.

18. *Essential Oils Desk Reference*, complied by Essential Science Publishing, 3rd printing, May 2000, 1, 120–21.

19. John D. B. Featherstone, MSc, PhD, "The Science and Practice of Caries Prevention," *JADA*, vol. 131, July 2000, 887–99.

20. D. Sambunjak, et al., 2011, ibid.

21. Sigard P. Ramford, LDS, MS, PhD, and Major M. Ash, Jr., BS, DDS, MS, *Periodontology and Periodontics.* WB Saunders Company, Philadelphia, PA, 1979, 23–26, 65–70.

22. Thomas E. Rams and Jorgen Slots, "Local Delivery of Antimicrobial Agents in the Periodontal Pocket," *Periodontology 1996*, vol. 10, no. 1, 139–59.

23. J. A. Aas et al., 2005, ibid., 5721–32.

24. Surgeon's General Report on Oral Health Finds Profound Disparities in Nation's Population, NIDCR News (National Institute of Dental & Craniofacial Research, National Institute of Health), May 25, 2000, Bethesda, MD.

25. YouTube: 1950's Howdy Doody Sees a Dentist PSA.

26. Guy Giacopazzi III, DDS, "But All I Want Is a Cleaning," *Viewpoint ADA News*, May 15, 1989.

27. Pamela Marogliano-Muniz, DMD, "Alternatives to Floss: A Review of Sunstar Gum's Soft-pick Advanced," August 22, 2016, *Dentistry IQ*.

28. Nancy W. Burkhart, BSDH, EdD, "Oral Oil Pulling," *RDH Magazine*, May 2014.

29. Nancy W. Burkhart, BSDH, EdD, 2014, ibid.

30. W. Galvan et al., "Periodontal Effects of 0.25% Sodium Hypochlorite Twice-weekly Oral Rinse. A Pilot Study," *J Periodontal Res*, December 14, 2013, vol. 49, no. 6, 696–702.

31. M. K. Bruch, "Toxicity and Safety of Topical Sodium Hypochlorite," *Contrib Nephrol*, 2007, vol. 154, 24–38.

32. Randal Eckert, et al., "Target Killing of Streptococcus Mutans by a Phero-mone-Guided 'Smart' Antimicrobial Peptide," *Antimicrobial Agents and Chemotherapy*, vol. 50, no. 11, November 2006.

33. P. Milgram et al., "Mutans Streptococci Dose Response to Xylitol Chewing Gum," *J Dental Research*, vol. 85, no. 2, 2006, 177–81.

34. E. C. Reynolds, "Remineralization of Enamel Subsurface Lesions by Casein Phosphopeptide-stabilized Calcium Phosphate Solutions," *J Dent Res*, September, 1997, vol. 76, no. 9, 1587–95.

35. A. Kiet, MD, MPH, et al., "Xylitol, Sweeteners, and Dental Caries." *Pediatric Dentistry*, 2006, vol. 28, no. 2, 154–63.

36. Ibid.

37. Ibid.

38. Y. Li and D. W. Caufield, "The Fidelity of Initial Acquisition of Mutans Streptococci by Infants from their Mothers," *J Dent Res*, vol. 74, no. 2: February 1995, 681–85.

39. T. Oku and S. Nakamura, "Threshold for Transitory Diarrhea Induced by Ingestion of Xylitol and Lactitol in Young Male and Female Adults," *J Nutr Sci Vitaminol* (Tokyo), February 2007, vol. 53, no. 1: 13–20.

40. Ahna Brutlay, DVM, MS, DABVT, "Xylitol Toxicity in Dogs," VCA Animal Hospital, vcahospitals.com.

41. E. Newbrun et al., "Bactericidal Action of Bicarbonate Ion on Selected Periodontal Pathogenic Microorganisms," *J Periodontol*, November 1984, vol. 55, no. 11, 658–67.

42. Brian Novy, DDS, 2007, ibid.

43. Brian Novy, DDS, 2007, ibid.

44. William G. Shafer, BS, DDS, MS, et al., Dental Caries chapter in *A Textbook of Oral Pathology*, 3rd edition, 1974, WB Saunders Company, Philadelphia, PA, 366–432.

45. William G. Shafer, BS, DDS, MS, 1974, ibid., 711.

46. ADA, "Fluoridation Facts," 2005.

47. William J. Hirzy, MD, PhD, "Why EPA's Headquarters Professionals Union Opposes Fluoridation," 1998, National Federation of Federal Employees, Local 2050.

48. John A. Yiamouyiannis, PhD, "Water Fluoridation & Tooth Decay: Result from the 1986-1987 National Survey of U.S. School Children," *Fluoride: J Inter Society for Fluoride Research*, April 1990, vol 23, no. 2, 55–67.

49. B. T. Amaechi, et al., "Remineralization of Artificial Enamel Lesions by Theobromine," *Caries Research*, April 24, 2013, vol. 47, no. 5, 399–405.

50. A. Moritz, et al., "Treatment of Periodontal Pockets with a Diode Laser," *Lasers Surg Med*, 1998, vol. 22, no. 5, 302–11.

CHAPTER 2. FROM OUR MIND TO OUR MOUTH: HOLISTIC DENTISTRY AND THE MEDICAL HEALTH CONNECTION

1. Jeremy Hugh Brown, "Sailor's Scurvy Before and After James Lind—A Reassessment," *Nutrition Review*, vol. 67, no. 6: 315–32.

2. Michael L. Barnett, DDS, "The Oral-systemic Disease Connection," *JADA*, October, 2006, vol 137, Supplement 2, S5–S6.

3. Bill Landers, "How Fast Do the Bacteria in Your Mouth Grow?" *Oratalk*, Fall 2006, 3.

4. Jerry Tennant, MD, MD(H), PScD, "Healing Is Voltage: Cancer's On/Off Switches :Polarity," 2015, San Bernardino, CA, www.tennantinstitute.com.

5. Michael Gerber, MD, HMD, ISOM Vancouver, Canada, review of "Oxidative Stress: Common Denominator of Chronic Degenerative Disease," reported in "Monthly Miracles: Cancer Revolutions," *Townsend Letter*, August/September 2016, 101–4.

6. H. Stan McGuff, DDS et al., "Maxillary Osteosarcoma Associated with a Dental Implant," *JADA*, August 2008, vol. 139, no. 8, 1052–59.

7. Pablo Galindo-Moreno, DDS, PhD, et al., "Multifocal Oral Melanoacanthoma and Melanotic Macula in a Patient After Dental Implant Surgery," *JADA*, July 2011, vol. 142, no. 7, 817–24.

8. IAOMT, "2016 Fact Sheet on Human Health Risks from Dental Amalgam Mercury fillings," Comprehensive Review of Dental Mercury, www.iaomt.org.

9. U.S. Food and Drug Administration, Department of Health and Human Services, "Final Rule: Classifying Dental Amalgam," online press release, July 28, 2009, www.fda.gov/Newsevents/Newsroom/PressAnnouncements/ucm173992.htm.

10. IAOMT, 2016 Fact Sheet, ibid.

11. *Casarett and Doull's "Toxicology: The Basic Science of Poisons,"* 5th edition, McGraw Hill, New York, NY, 1996.

12. Boyd Haley, PhD, "GCF Components," Affinity Labeling Technologies, Inc., University of Kentucky, Lexington, KY, www.altcorp.com.

13. Physician's Desk Reference, 63rd edition, 2008, Physician's Desk Reference, Inc., Montvale, NJ, www.PDR.net, "Lidocaine Viscous Solutions."

14. Walter Jess Clifford, MS, "Clifford Materials Reactivity Testing, Summary— At A Glance," www.ccrlab.com.

15. Abby F. Fleisch, et al., "Bisphenol A and Related Compounds in Dental Materials," *Pediatrics*, October 2010, vol. 126, no. 4.

16. David C. Kennedy, DDS, IAOMT's "Policy Position on Ingested Fluoride and Fluoridation," January 2003, www.iaomt.org.

17. FDA News Release, "FDA Issues Final Rule on Safety and Effectiveness of Antibacterial Soaps," September 2, 2016.

18. Bloomberg, "Cancer-linked Colgate Total Ingredient Suggests Flaws in FDA Approval Process," 2014, www.bloomberg.com.

19. William G. Shafer, DDS, MS, et al. 1974, ibid., 360–432.

20. William Randall Kellas, PhD, and Andrea Sharon Dworkin, ND, *Thriving in a Toxic World: Tools for Flourishing in the 21st Century,* Quality Books, Inc. 1996, 235, 245, 349–53.

21. Barry Sears, MD, *The Anti-Inflammation Zone: Reversing the Silent Epidemic That's Destroying Our Health,* HarperCollins Publishers, New York, NY, 2005, 12.

22. Jeremy Mikolai, ND, "Vascular Biology, Endothelial Function, and Natural Rehabilitation: Part 2: Oxidative and Nitrosative Stress," *Townsend Letter,* June 2014, 74–81.

CHAPTER 3. NUTRITION: HOW "FRIENDLY"
FOODS AFFECT YOUR TEETH AND GUMS

1. Udo Erasmus, *Fats that Heal, Fats that Kill*, 1993, 11th printing, Alive Books, Burnaby, BC, Canada, 6, 73–74.

2. Weston Price, DDS, ibid., xv, xvi, 1, 300, 472, 474–75.

3. Erasmus, Udo, 1993, ibid., 43–51.

4. Barry Sears, MD, 2005, ibid., 81.

5. Erasmus, Udo, 1993, ibid., 259.

6. Erasmus, Udo, 1993, ibid.

7. William Randall Kellas, PhD and Andrea Sharon Dworkin, 1996, ibid., 249.

8. William R. Kellas, PhD et al., 1996, ibid., 249–56.

9. William R. Kellas, PhD et al., 1996, ibid., 264–65.

10. William R. Kellas, PhD, et al., 1996, ibid., 259.

11. Barry Sears, MD, 2005, ibid., 63, 71, 73.

12. Barry Sears, MD, 2005, ibid., 63–64.

13. William R. Kellas, PhD et al., 1996, ibid., 318, 250, 260.

14. Erasmus, Udo, 1993, ibid., 227–30.

15. William R. Kellas, PhD et al., 1996, ibid., 259–60.

16. Barry Sears, MD, 2005, ibid., 50–56.

17. Barry Sears, MD, 2005, ibid, 50–56.

18. William R. Kellas, PhD et al., 1996, ibid., 305–6.

19. William R. Kellas, PhD et al., 1996, ibid., 294.

20. Vitamin D*action, *Grassroots Health*, www.grassrootshealth.net.

21. William R. Kellas, PhD et al., 1996, ibid., 309–10.

22. William R. Kellas, PhD et al., 1996, ibid., 312.

23. William R. Kellas, PhD et al., 1996, ibid., 311.

24. William R. Kellas, PhD et al., 1996, ibid., 283–306, 309–33.

25. Carolyn Mein, DC, *Different Bodies Different Diets: The Revolutionary 25 Body Type System*, 2001, HarperCollins Publishers, Inc., New York, NY.

26. Dr. Barry Sears, 2005, ibid.

27. Ed Group III, DC, ND, DACBN, DABFM, *The Green Body Cleanse: How to Cleanse Your Body and House of Harmful Toxins Using Organic Methods*, 2009, Global Healing Center, LP, Houston, TX, book and website, www.globalhealingcenter.com.

28. Weston Price, DDS, 1997, ibid., 378.

29. Weston Price, DDS, 1997, ibid., 421–22, 442–43.

30. Jonathan V. Wright, MD, IAOMT lecture handout, *Nutritional Supplementation Suggested Protocols*, March 2003.

31. Brian Novy, DDS, 2007, ibid.

32. Warden H. Noble, DDS, MS, MSED, et al., "Sports Drinks and Dental Erosion," *CDA Journal,* vol. 39, no. 4, April 2011, 233–34.

33. Randy Q. Ligh, DDS, MA, et al., "The Effects of Nutrition and Diet on Dental Structure Integrity," *CDA Journal*, vol. 39, no. 4, April 2011, 243–45.

34. William R. Kellas, PhD et al., 1996, ibid., 314–15, 325–26.

CHAPTER 4. CHAKRAS, MERIDIANS, AND THE HEART: HOW MATTER AND ENERGY AFFECT YOUR ORAL HEALTH

1. Bruce Lipton, PhD, *"The Biology of Belief: Unleashing the Power of Consciousness, Matter & Miracles,"* 2008, Hay House, Inc., 155.

2. Eden Alexander, MD, "Living in a Mindful Universe: A Neurosurgeon's Journey into the Heart of Consciousness," Rodale Inc., 2017, 53, 60–61, 66–67.

3. Bruce Lipton, PhD, 2008, ibid., 68–71.

4. James Arthur Ray, *Harmonic Wealth: The Secret of Attracting the Life You Want,"* Hyperion, NY, 2008, 2–3, 10, 43–47.

5. Masaru Emoto, 2002, "Messages from Water," *HADO Kyoikusha,* Tokyo, Japan.

6. David R. Hawkins, MD, 1998, *Power vs. Force: The Hidden Determinants of Human Behavior,* Veritas Publishing, Sedona, AZ, 52–53.

7. Edward F. Group III, DC, PhD, November 2, 2002, "Cellular Consciousness & Disease: Has Science Been Wrong?" lecture handout: "Dr. Group's Degeneration Disease Model and Solution."

8. Amit Goswami, PhD, *"God Is Not Dead: What Quantum Physics Tells Us About Our Origins and How We Should Live,"* 2008, Hampton Roads Publishing Company, Charlottesville, VA, 17.

9. Amit Goswami, PhD, *How Quantum Activism Can Save Civilization,* 2011, Hampton Roads Publishing Company, Inc, Charlottesville, VA, 4–5.

CHAPTER 5. STRESS BUSTERS: A ROADMAP TO INNER PEACE

1. Robert M. Williams, MA, 2000, *Psych-K: The Missing Peace in Your Life,* Spirit 2000, Inc. Publications, Memphis, Tennessee, 113–18.

2. Prime One: Adaptogenic Formula, SABA for you. For life, Oklahoma City, OK, www.sabaforlife.com.

3. R. C. Wiener PhD, et al., "Association of Tooth Loss and Depression and Anxiety." At the AADR 43rd Annual Meeting, March 20, 2014.

4. Robert M. Williams, MA, 2000, ibid., 113–18.

5. Clayton A. Chan, DDS, FICCMO, August 30, 2002, *"The Neuromuscular Dentist,"* Lecture at Occlusion I: Practical Occlusion for the Progressive Practice, Las Vegas Institute, Las Vegas, NV.

6. Tiffany Snow, DD, *Psychic Gifts in the Christian Life: Tools to Connect,* San Marcos, CA, Spirit Journey Books, 2003, 4.

7. Tiffany Snow, DD, *God's Workbook: Shifting into Light,* San Marcos, CA, Spirit Journey Books, 2007, 254–55.

8. Derek M. Watson et al., "Killing the Victim: Before the Victim Kills You," 1996, Mashiyach Press, Santa Rosa, CA, 27–30, 159, 231.

9. Tiffany Snow, DD, 2007, ibid., 5, 271–73.

10. S. A. Lawrence, DDS, *"Victorious Living Through Self-Government"* (Masters of Canonical Jurisprudence diss., Saint Mark Seminary and College, 2010), 51.

11. S. A. Lawrence, 2010, ibid., 18.

12. S. A. Lawrence, 2010, ibid., 41.

13. S. A. Lawrence, 2010, ibid., 101–108.

14. S. A. Lawrence, 2010, ibid., 51–53.

CHAPTER 6. LOVE AND WELLNESS

1. David R. Hawkins, MD, PhD, 1998, ibid., 52–53.

2. Connie and Alan Higley, *Reference Guide for Essential Oils*, Abundant Health, 2006, 10th ed.

3. Derek M. Watson et al., 1996, ibid.

4. Dean Schrock, PhD, *Why Love Heals: Body-Mind-Spirit Medicine*, Heartfelt Intent Publishing, Eagle Point, OR, 2009, 162, 243.

5. Forbes, Harvard study, 2014, *Top 10 Common Toxins Causing ADHD and Autism.*

6. Tiffany Snow, DD, ibid., 75, 151–58.

7. Dean Schrock, PhD, 2009, ibid., 80.

8. Tiffany Snow, DD, 2007, ibid., 75, 151–58.

9. Tiffany Snow, DD, 2007, ibid., 103, 300.

10. Tiffany Snow, DD, 2007, ibid., 119, 146, 177.

CHAPTER 7. THE BALANCE OF THE UNIVERSE AND YOUR TEETH

1. Stephen A. Lawrence, DDS, 2010, ibid., 9.

2. Tiffany Snow, DD, 2007, ibid., 135, 213.

3. Tiffany Snow, DD, 2007, ibid., 254.

CHAPTER 8. LOVE AND HEALING

1. T. Snow, DD, 2006, *Forward From the Mind: Distant Healing, Bilocation, Medical Intuition & Prayer in a Quantum World*, San Marcos, CA, Spirit Journey Books, 223–24.

2. M. Emoto, 2002, ibid.

3. Eber Alexander, MD, 2017, ibid., chapters 13 and 14.

4. T. Snow, DD and B. Clark, 2007, ibid., 254–55.

5. T. Snow, DD, *The Power of Divine: A Healer's Guide,* Spirit Journey Books, San Marcos, CA, 2004, 125.

6. A. Goswami, PhD, *How Quantum Activism Can Save Civilization.* Hampton Roads Publishing Company, Inc., Charlottesville, VA, 2011, xiv–xv, 5.

7. Ibid., 2011, 42–43.

8. Ibid., 2011, 138.

9. Eben Alexander, MD, 2017, ibid., 30, 33, 60, 66.

10. A. Goswami, PhD., 2011, ibid., 159.

11. T. Snow, DD, 2003, *Psychic Gifts in the Christian Life: Tools to Connect.* San Marcos, CA: Spirit Journey Books, 47–69.

12. T. Snow, DD, 2003, ibid., 50–53.

13. Ibid., 2003, 56.

14. Ibid., 2003, 65–66.

Bibliography

Aas, J. A., et al. "Defining the Normal Bacterial Flora of the Oral Cavity," *J Clin Microbiol*, November 2005, vol. 43, no. 11: 5721–32.

ADA, "Fluoridation Facts," 2005.

Adler, Christina J., et al. "Sequencing Ancient Calcified Dental Plaque Shows Changes in Oral Microbiota with Dietary Shifts of the Neolithic and Industrial Revolutions," *Nature Genetic*, 2013, vol. 45, 450–55. DOI: 10.1038/ng.2536.

Alexander, Eben, MD. *Living in a Mindful Universe: A Neurosurgeon's Journey into the Heart of Consciousness*, Rodale Inc., 2017.

Amaechi, B. T., et al. "Remineralization of Artificial Enamel Lesions by Theobromine," *Caries Research*, April 24, 2013, vol. 47, no. 5, 399–405.

Anderson, Maxwell, DDS, MS, Med. et al. "Modern Management of Dental Caries: The Cutting Edge Is Not the Dental Bur," *JADA*, June 1993, vol. 124, no. 6, 36–44.

Barnett, Michael L., DDS. "The Oral-systemic Disease Connection," *JADA*, October 2006, vol. 137, supplement 2, S5–S6.

Bloomberg. "Cancer-linked Colgate Total Ingredient Suggests Flaws in FDA Approval Process," 2014, www.bloomberg.com.

Brown, Jeremy Hugh. "Sailor's Scurvy Before and After James Lind—A Reassessment," *Nutrition Review*, vol. 67, no. 6: 315–32.

Bruch, M. K. "Toxicity and Safety of Topical Sodium Hypochlorite," *Contrib Nephrol*, 2007, vol. 154, 24–38.

Brutlay, Ahna, DVM, MS, DABVT. "Xylitol Toxicity in Dogs." VCA Animal Hospital, vcahospitals.com.

Burkhart, Nancy W., BSDH, EdD. "Oral Oil Pulling," *RDH Magazine*, May 2014.

Casarett and Doull's *Toxicology: The Basic Science of Poisons*. 5th edition, McGraw Hill, New York, NY, 1996.

Chan, Clayton A., DDS, FICCMO. August 30, 2002, "*The Neuromuscular Dentist,*" Lecture at Occlusion I: Practical Occlusion for the Progressive Practice, Las Vegas Institute, Las Vegas, NV.

Clifford, Walter Jess, MS. "Clifford Materials Reactivity Testing: Summary—At a Glance," www.ccrlab.com.

Costerton, J. W., and Philip S. Stewart. "Battling Biofilms," *Emerging Trends in Oral Care*, Scientific American, Inc., New York, NY, 2002, 6–12.

Davey, A. L., and A. H. Roger. "Multiple Types of the Bacterium Streptococcus Mutans in the Human Mouth and Their Intra-family Transmission," *Arch Oral Biol*, 1984, vol. 29, no. 6, 453–60.

Eckert, Randal, et al. "Target Killing of Streptococcus Mutans by a Pheromone-Guided 'Smart' Antimicrobial Peptide," *Antimicrobial Agents and Chemotherapy*, vol. 50, no. 11, November 2006.

Emoto, Masaru. 2002. "The Message from Water," *Hado Kyoikusha*.

Erasmus, Udo. *Fats that Heal, Fats that Kill*, 11th printing. Alive Books, Burnaby, BC, Canada, 1993.

Essential Oils Desk Reference, complied by Essential Science Publishing, 3rd printing, May 2000, 1, 120–21.

Featherstone, John, DB, MSc, PhD. "The Science and Practice of Caries Prevention," *JADA*, vol 131, (7), July 2000, 887–99.

Fleisch, Abby F., et al. "Bisphenol A and Related Compounds in Dental Materials," *Pediatrics*, October 2010, vol. 126, no. 4.

Forbes, Harvard study, 2014, "Top 10 Common Toxins Causing ADHD and Autism."

Galindo-Moreno, Pablo, DDS, PhD, et al. "Multifocal Oral Melanoacanthoma and Melanotic Macula in a Patient After Dental Implant Surgery," *JADA*, July 2011, vol 142, no. 7, 817–24.

Galvin. W., et al., "Periodontal Effects of 0.25% Sodium Hypochlorite Twice Weekly Oral Rinse. A Pilot Study," *J Periodontal Res.,* December 14, 2013, vol. 49, no. 6, 696–702.

Gerber, Michael, MD, HMD, ISOM Vancouver, Canada, review of "Oxidative Stress: Common Denominator of Chronic Degenerative Disease," reported in "Monthly Miracles: Cancer Revolutions," *Townsend Letter*, August/September 2016, 101–104.

Giacopazzi III, Guy, DDS. "But All I Want Is a Cleaning," *Viewpoint ADA News*, May 15, 1989.

Goswami, Amit, PhD. *God Is Not Dead: What Quantum Physics Tells Us About Our Origins and How We Should Live,* Hampton Roads Publishing Company, Charlottesville, VA, 2008, 17.

———. *How Quantum Activism Can Save Civilization*, Charlottesville, VA: Hampton Roads Publishing Company, Inc., 2011, xiv–xv, 4–5, 159.

Grassroots Health, "Vitamin D*action," www.grassrootshealth.net.

Group III, Ed, DC, ND, DACBN, DABFM. "*The Green Body Cleanse: How to Cleanse Your Body and House of Harmful Toxins Using Organic Methods,*" 2009, Global Healing Center, LP, Houston, TX, book and website, www.globalhealing center.com.

———. November 2, 2002, "Cellular Consciousness & Disease: Has Science Been Wrong?" Lecture Handout: "Dr. Group's Degeneration Disease Model and Solution."

Haley, Boyd, PhD. "GCF Components," Affinity Labeling Technologies, Inc., University of Kentucky, Lexington, KY, www.altcorp.com.

Hawkins, David R., MD. "*Power vs. Force: The Hidden Determinants of Human Behavior*," Veritas Publishing, Sedona, AZ, 1998.

Higley, Connie and Alan. *Reference Guide for Essential Oils,* 10 ed., *Abundant Health,* 2006.

Hirzy, William J., MD, PhD. "Why EPA's Headquarters Professionals Union Opposes Fluoridation," 1998, National Federation of Federal Employees, Local 2050.

Houte, Juan. "Role of Micro-organisms in the Caries Etiology," *J Dent Res*, March 1994, vol. 73, no. 3: 672–91.

International Association of Oral Medicine and Toxicology (IAOMT), "2016 Fact Sheet on Human Health Risks from Dental Amalgam Mercury Fillings."

Ioannidis, John P. A. August 2005, "Why Most Published Findings Are False," *Plos Medicine,* 1–10, plosmedicine.org/article/info:doi/10.1371/journal.pmed.0020124.

Kellas, William Randall, PhD, and Andrea Sharon Dworkin, ND. *Thriving in a Toxic World: Tools for Flourishing in the 21st Century*, Quality Books, Inc. 1996.

Kennedy, David C., DDS. IAOMT's "Policy Position on Ingested Fluoride and Fluoridation," January 2003, www.iaomt.org.

Kiet A., MD, MPH, et al. "Xylitol, Sweeteners, and Dental Caries." *Pediatric Dentistry*, 2006, vol. 28, no. 2, 154–63.

Landers, Bill. "How Fast Do Bacteria in Your Mouth Grow?" *Oratalk*, Fall, 2006, vol. 3.

Lawrence, Stephen A. "Victorious Living Through Self-Government." M.A. thesis, Saint Mark Seminary and College, 2010.

Li, Y., and C. W. Caufield. "The Fidelity of Initial Acquisition of Mutans Streptococci by Infants from their Mothers," *J Dent Res*, February 1995, vol. 74, no. 2, 681–85.

Ligh, Randy Q., DDS, MA, et al. The Effects of Nutrition and Diet on Dental Structure Integrity, *CDA Journal*, April 2011, vol. 39, no. 4, 243–45.

Lipton, Bruce, PhD. "The Biology of Belief: Unleashing the Power of Consciousness, Matter & Miracles," Hay House, Inc., 2008.

Marogliano-Muniz, Pamela, DMD. "Alternatives to Floss: A Review of Sunstar Gum's Soft-pick Advanced," August 22, 2016, *Dentistry IQ*.

McGuff, H. Stan, DDS, et al. "Maxillary Osteosarcoma Associated with a Dental Implant," *JADA*, August 2008, vol. 139, no. 8, 1052–59.

Mein, Carolyn, DC. *Different Bodies Different Diets: The Revolutionary 25 Body Type System,* 2001, HarperCollins Publishers, Inc., New York, NY.

Mikolai, Jeremy, MD. "Vascular Biology, Endothelial Function, and Natural Rehabilitation; Part 2: Oxidative and Nitrosative Stress," *Townsend Letter*, June 2014, 74–81.

Milgram, P., et al. "Mutans Streptococci Dose Response to Xylitol Chewing Gum," *J Dental Research*, vol. 85, no. 2, 2006, 177–81.

Moritz, A., et al. "Treatment of Periodontal Pockets with a Diode Laser," *Lasers Surg Med,* 1998, 22 (5), 302–11.

Newbrun, E., et al. "Bactericidal Action of Bicarbonate Ion on Selected Periodontal Pathogenic Microorganisms," *J Periodontol*, November 1984, 55 (11), 658–667.

Newbrun, Ernest. 1989. *Cariology*, Quintessence Publishing Company, Microflora, 44–75.

Noble, Warren H., DDS, MS, MSED, et al. "Sports Drinks and Dental Erosion," *CDA Journal*, vol 39, no 4, April 2011, 233–34.

Novy, Brian, DDS. CEA Dental Convention lecture, *"The Cutting Edge of Caries Management,"* November 2007.

Oku, T. and S. Nakamura. "Threshold for Transitory Diarrhea Induced by Ingestion of Xylitol and Lactitol in Young Male and Female Adults," *J Nutr Sci Vitaminol* (Tokyo), February 2007, 53 (1): 13–20.

Overman, Pamela R., RDH, MS. "Biofilm: A New View of Plaque," *J Contemporary Dental Practice*, vol 1, no 3, Summer issue, 2000, 1–8.

Physician's Desk Reference, 63rd ed. 2008, published by Physician's Desk Reference, Inc., Montvale, NJ, www.PDR.net, "Lidocaine Viscous Solutions."

Price, Weston, DDS. *Nutrition and Physical Degeneration*, 1997, 6th ed., Price-Pottenger Nutrition Foundation, La Mesa, CA, xv, xvi, 1, 300, 378, 421–22, 442–43, 472, 474–75.

Prime One: Adaptogenic Formula. *SABA for you. For life*. Oklahoma City, OK. www .sabaforlife.com.

Ramford, Sigard P., LDS, MS, PhD, and Major M. Ash, Jr., BS, DDS, MS. *Periodontology and Periodontics*. W.B. Saunders Company, Philadelphia, PA, 1979, 23–26, 65–70.

Rams, Thomas E. and Jorgen Slots. "Local Delivery of Antimicrobial Agents in the Periodontal Pocket," *Periodontology*, 2000; vol 10, (1), 1996, 139–59.

Ray, James Arthur. 2008. "Harmonic Wealth: The Secret of Attracting the Life You Want," Hyperion, NY, 2–3, 10, 43–47.

Reynolds, E. C. "Remineralization of Enamel Subsurface Lesions by Casein Phosphopeptide-stabilized Calcium Phosphate Solutions," *J Dent Res*, September, 1997, 76, (9), 1587–95.

Sambunjak D., et al. "Flossing for the Management of Periodontal Diseases and Dental Caries in Adults," *Cochrane Database Syst Rev*, 2011 (12): CDOO8829, Pub 2.

Schrock, Dean, PhD. *Why Love Heals: Mind-Body-Spirit Medicine*, Heartfelt Intent Publishing, Eagle Point, OR, 2009, 162, 243.

———. *Why Love Heals: Mind-Body-Spirit Medicine*, Eagle Point, OR, Heartfelt Intent Publications, 118–20.

Sears, Barry, MD. *The Anti-Inflammation Zone*, 2005, Harper Collins Publishers, New York, NY, 1x–4, 50–56, 63–64, 71, 73, 81.

Shafer, William G., BS, DDS, MS, et al. Dental Caries chapter in: *A Textbook of Oral Pathology*, 3rd ed., 1974, WB Saunders Company, Philadelphia, PA, 366–432.

Snow, Tiffany, DD. *God's Workbook*, Spirit Journey Books, San Marcos, CA, 2007, 75, 103, 119, 135, 146, 151–58, 177, 254–55, 300.

———. *"The Power of Divine: A Healer's Guide, Tapping into the Miracle."* San Marcos, CA: Spirit Journey Books, 2004.

————. *Forward From the Mind: Distant Healing, Bilocation, Medical Intuition & Prayer in a Quantum World*, San Marcos, CA: Spirit Journey Books, 2006.

————. *Psychic Gifts in the Christian Life: Tools to Connect.* San Marcos, CA: Spirit Journey Books, 2003.

Southward, Ken, DDS, FAGD. "The Systemic Theory of Dental Caries," *General Dentistry*, September/October 2011, vol 59, no. 5, 367–73.

Steinmen, Ralph, DDS, MS, and John Leonora, PhD. *Dentinal Fluid Transport*, Loma Linda University Press, 2004.

Surgeon's General Report on "Oral Health Finds Profound Disparities in Nation's Population," *NIDCR News* (National Institute of Dental & Craniofacial Research), National Institute of Health, May 25, 2000, Bethesda, MD.

Tadinada, A., et al. "The Evolution of a Tooth Brush: From Antiquity to Present—A Mini Review," 2015, 2 (4) 00055DOI: 10.15406/jdhodt 2015.0200055. *J of Dental Health*, Oral Disorders & Therapy.

Tennant, Jerry, MD, MD(H), PScD. "Healing Is Voltage: Cancer's On/Off Switches-Polarity," 2015, San Bernardino, CA, www.tennantinstitute.com.

U.S. Food and Drug Administration, Department of Health and Human Services, "Final Rule: Classifying Dental Amalgam," online press release, July 28, 2009, www.fda.gov/Newsevents/Newsroom/PressAnnouncements/ucm173992.htm.

Watson, Derek M., et al. *Killing the Victim Before It Kills You*, Mashiyach Press, Santa Rosa, CA, 1996.

Wiener, R. C., et al. March 20, 2014, "Association of Tooth Loss and Depression and Anxiety." AADR, 43rd Annual Meeting.

Williams, Robert M., MA. *Psych-K: The Missing Peace in Your Life.* 113–18. Spirit 2000, Inc. Publications, Memphis, Tennessee, 2000.

Wright, Jonathan V., MD. IAOMT Lecture Handout, *Nutritional Supplementation Suggested Protocols*, March 2003.

Yiamouyiannis, John A., PhD. "Water Fluoridation & Tooth Decay: Results from the 1986–1987 National Survey of U.S. School Children," *Fluoride: J. Inter Society for Fluoride Research,* April 1990, vol. 23, no. 2, 55–67.

Index

acids: ascorbic, 53; attacks of, 26,80; essential amino, 72–74, ; fatty, 71; folic, *84*; from food and drinks, 80–81, *85*; hexuronic, 53; nutrition and, 80–81; omega 3 fatty, *84*; para-aminobenzoic, 62

active Ca PO4 (ACP), 39

activator X, 79

acupuncture, 66, 100; meridians in, 57,*58*

The ADA Council on Dental Therapeutics, 37

adrenal cortex, 53

adrenal glands, 122

AK. *See* applied kinesiology

Alanine, 73

alkaline phosphate, 61

allergies, 60–61

allopathic medicine, 3

aluminum, 61

Alzheimer's disease, *52*,*54*, 60–61

amino acids, essential, 72–74,

anesthetics: in dentistry, 2, 62–63; as poison, 49

antibiotics, resistance to, 60

antibodies, 61

antioxidants, 9, 20

anxiety, 108–10

applied kinesiology (AK), 94

Arginine, 41, 73, 85

Arsenic, 122

arthritis, 2, 49, *52,* 54, 61

ascorbic acid, 53

authentic holistic dentistry, 1, 5, 9, 133

autism spectrum disorders, 60

autoimmune system, 57, 60

Ayurvedic medicine, 36

bacteria: bad, 96, 117; diversity of, 13–15; food for, 28; good, 117, 129; history of, 13–15; host-mediated, 51; in root canals, 56; oral, 13

baking soda, 41, 43; in toothpaste, 119

BANA hydrolysis, 19

barbers, in early dentistry, 50

Bellinger, David C., PhD, MSc, 122

benzocaine, 62

beryllium, 61

biochemistry, in dentistry, 65

biofilm, 14, *16, 18, 23*; colonies, 31, 32; irrigation and, 29, 30–31; theory, 19, 50

biology, of dentistry, 51,

Bisphenol A, 63

Black Plague, 26
Bleach, *see* dilute bleach
bleeding gums, friable, 53
Blessed Tiffany, 123
blessings, 94, 130–31,139–40
body: emotional, 1, 6, 105, 147; physical, 1, 6, 147; spiritual, 1, 6, 133–34, 147
Body Type diet, 78
BPA, 4
Brekhman, Israel, Dr., 108
bridges, 9, 50, 59
bruising, 53
brushing, *see* toothbrushing
bugs, *see* bacteria

cacao extract, 45
calcium, 15, 20, 43, 51, 77, 83, *84, 87*; levels of, 54
cancer, 44, *52*; gum disease and, 54; implants and, 2, 49, 57
candida, 60
CANI. *See* Constant and Never Ending Improvement
carbohydrates, 74–75
caries, dental. *See* cavities
Caries Management Protocol, 41–43
carrageen, 122
casein phosphopeptide (CCP), 39
catcher, 123
cavities: 2; biology of, 51, *52, 54*; formation of, 14–15, *17*, 17–19, 80; gut health and, 20; history of, 12–13; primary cause of, 20; reverse, 2, 41–43, 82–83; strep mutans and, 14; sugar and, 20
central nervous system, damage to, 44
chakras, exploring, 98–99, *99*
chemistry, in dentistry , 59–60
chi, 100
Chinese, licorice root 38; medicine, 57; meridian system, 100
chiropath, 133
chiropractor, craniosacral, 66

chronic illnesses, 2, 49, 136; gum disease and, 54
chronic inflammation: oxidative stress and, 67; stress and, 108
church, 142
cleaning, microsonic, 19
Clifford Reactivity Test, 63
Closys, 25
co-create, 104, 123, 141
Coenzyme Q10, 83, *84*
colloidal silver protocol, 43
Constant and Never Ending Improvement (CANI), 7
craniosacral chiropractor, 66
crowns, dental fillings and, *55,* 60

dementia, senile, 61
dental anesthetics, 2, 49, 62–63
dental caries, management protocol for, 41–43
dental cleanings, 31–33, 42, 67–68
dental fillings, crowns and, 60
dental healthcare, 11; action list for, 145; adjunctive therapies and, 43; anxiety affecting, 109–10; archeological records for, 13; brief history of, *50,* 50–51; brushing for, 19, 23–28; bugs, biofilm, and balance in, 14–19, *15, 16, 17*; cavities and gum disease history in, 12–13; dental caries management, 41–43; depression affecting, 109–10; diet influencing, 12–13; different cultures influencing, 12; disease vs health, 19–20, *21*; food and, 28–33, *29*; hygienist cleanings and, 31–33; indents affecting, 112–13; irrigating teeth and gums in, 28–31, *29*; jaw problems affecting, 111–12; oil pulling and, 36; optimal health and vitality in, 12; psychoimmunological factors affecting, 110–11; teeth longevity and, 21–22; tooth anatomy in, *29*; fighting tooth decay , 38–41; tooth loss affecting, 109–10; tooth

picking and, 33–35, *34*; victimization and, 113–16

Dental Herb Company, 25, 119

dental hygiene products, chemicals in, 64–65

dental implants, cancer and, 2, 49, 57–59, 100

dental plaque, *16*

dentistry: anesthetics in, 2, 49, 62–63; biochemistry in, 65; biology of, 51, *52*; chemistry of, 59–60; evidence-based, 3, 5; fear-based, *4*; holistic, 1, 3; metals in, 61; minimally invasive, 47

Dentiva lozenges, 39, 42, 46, 145

depression, 60, 109–10; from stress, 108

diabetes, 2, 49, 52, 54

diet: body type, 78, 146; dental healthcare and, 12–13; organic foods for, 128; poor, 20; of processed foods, 128–29; recommended, 78–79; SAD, 12, 72; universe balance and, 128–29

dilute bleach mouthrinse, 37, 43

disease, 3, 136

dissolving power: drinks, 85

The Divine Decrees, 131

Divine Spark, 89, 147

DNA probes, 19

DO. *See* osteopathic physicians

downward causation, 102–4, *103*

EAV, 100–1

Einstein, Albert, 91

electromotive forces (EMFs), 97, 101

emotional health, love and wellness and, 100, 120–21

Emoto, Masaru, Dr., 92, 137–38, 140

enamel, of tooth, 15, *29*

Endocal, 57

energy channels, 57, 100

energy levels, 91, 96–98, *97*, 111, 117–18, 138–39; everything is, 118, 138, 141; fear and, 121; with pets, 89, 127–28

entanglement, 89, 141

enzymes, 60–61

EPA, 44; fluoride 64

erosion, 85

Eramus, Udo, 72

essential amino acids. *See* amino acids, essential

essential oils, 25–26, 47; love and wellness and, 117; toothpaste and, *118, 119*

faith, 116

farming, 13

fasting, 142

fatigue, 60

fats, for nutrition, 71–72

Fats that Heal, Fats that Kill, 72

fatty acids, 71

FDA. *See* Federal Drug Administration

fear, 3, *4, 5, 100, 111, 114*; disease response to, 121; love and, 121–22, 136

Federal Drug Administration (FDA), toothpaste and, 49, 65

fillings, mercury, *4*, 60

Fischer, Emil, 39

flossing, 2, 50; alternatives to, 27; effectiveness of, 18–19, 27; research for, 27

flour, and sugar 13–15, 129

fluorapatite crystal, 44

fluoride, 50, 122; dangers of, 3, 64; toothpaste and, 117; toxicity of, 44–46

fluorosis, 45

folic acid, 83, *84*

forgiveness, 5, *93,* 123–24, 141, 143

fourth healing, 140

fractures, hip, 44

free radicals exposure, 20

free will: 120, 123, 139, action list for, 146; before birth, 138; concept of, 104, 137; fear and, 115, 137; protection, 139

fruit, citrus, 53

genetic damage, 45
gingivitis, 54
gluten, 81–82
God, 59, 114–16, 121, 123–25, 133, 134, 136, 142, 146–47
The Green Body Cleanse, 96
Group, Ed, Dr., 96, *97*
gum disease, 32, 46, 54, 82–83; biology of, 51; comorbidities of, 2; history of, 12–13, 19
gum pockets, 29, 54; fluids and, 30; healthy, 31; irrigation of, 19, 28–31
gums: health supplements for, 82, *84*; natural rebuilding of, 46; teeth and, 22–27

Hawkins, David, Dr., 94, 118
headaches, 60; from stress, 108–9
Healing Is Voltage, 56
healing touch practitioners, 67
hearing loss, 60
heart: disease, 2, 49; gum disease and, 54; human 123
herbs, 47
hexuronic acid, 53
Holes: drilling of, 9; teeth, 15,45
holistic dental model, 51, 92
holistic dentistry, 1, 3, 9; medical health connection and, 49–68, *50, 52, 58*; updates in, 2
holistic practitioners, 5, 66, 145
home, cooked meal 129
home water irrigation, instructions for, 38
Hooten, Earnest, Dr., 13
Hope, 116
Host, mediated 23, 49, 51, 96
Howdy Doody, 32
hydroxyapatite, 20; crystals, 43
hygienist, 19, 67–68
hypothalamus gland, 20, *21*, 43

IAOMT. *See* International Academy of Oral Medicine and Toxicology

immune system, 31; cells of, 53; investigation of, 49; mouth rinse and, 37; nutrition and, 33, 82–83, *84*; strong, 9, 22. *See also* autoimmune system
immunological blood reactivity test, 63
implants, 2, 9, 49; metal teeth, 57–59, 100
indent, 108, 112–13, 138–39
inflammation, chronic, 9, 49, 67
intention, 59, 104, 130
International Academy of Oral Medicine and Toxicology (IAOMT), 64, 82
iodine rinse, 24–25, 42
irrigation: biofilm colonies and, 28–31; home water instructions for, 38; of teeth and gums, 28–31, *29*

jaw problems, 111–12; from stress, 108

kale, 122
kidney disease, 60
Kirlian photography, 97–98, *98*

laser treatment, 19, 46
Levy, Thomas, MD, JD, 56
lidocaine, 62
Lind, James, 53
lollipops: 11–12; Loloz, 38, 42, 46, 145
love always wins, 6, 124, 135, 143, 147
love and healing: 109, 115–16, 121, 130, action list for, 146; balance and, 147; church and, 142; disease and, 136; fasting for, 142; fear and, 50, 107, 115, 121, 136; free will and, 137; free will protection and, 139; inter-connection and, 141; meditation for, 142; sacred spaces for, 142; self-protection and, 140–41; spiritual connections and, 141–42; spiritual frequencies in, 93–94, 138–39; spiritual toolkit for, 139–40, 142–43; water and life for, 137–38; your home and, 140–41

love and wellness: choosing, 5, 121–22, 126, 136; in dental products, 118; emotional health and, 120–21; energy levels and, 95, 117–18; essential oils and, 117, *118*; fear and, 121–22, 136; forgiveness and, 123–24; in homemade toothpaste, 119–20; lifelong fulfillment of, 126; in reducing stressors, 118; showing, 126; toothpaste and, 113, 117

love, water photo, *93*

lozenge, 39, 42

magnesium, 54, 60, 77, *84*

Makinen, Kauko, 40

malpractice, 33

Manganese, 122

Map of Consciousness, 94, *95*

massage, gentle gum, 35

maxillary osteosarcoma, 57

Mead, Margaret, 104

medicine, allopathic, 3; holistic, 66

meditation, 142

Mein, Carolyn, 78

melanoacanthoma, 59

melanotic macula, 59

memory loss, 60

mercury, 3; fillings, 4, 50, 59, 60

meridians: in acupuncture, 56–57; blocking of, 49

meridian systems, 58, 100

metallothionein, 60

metals, in dentistry, 59, 61

Methyl mercury, 122

microbiology, golden age of, 18

microscope: invention of, 18; phase contrast, 19, 36, 46; scanning electron, 19

microsonic cleaning, 19

milk, 74

minerals, essential, 77–78

MI Paste, 39, 42, 46, 145

miracles, be realistic expect, 139

mouth, chronic inflammation in, 49

mouth rinses: 26; dilute bleach, 37; effectiveness of, 18; instructions for, 37

multiple sclerosis, 60

naturopath, 66

neem, toothbrush, 24

neglect, supervised, 33

neurofibrillary tangles, 60

neuromuscular (NM) dentists, 111

Newtonian models of physics, 3, 90

niacin, 78, *84*

nickel, 3, 4, 61

NM. *See* neuromuscular dentists

Non-specific plaque hypotheses, 18

nutrients, essential, 69

nutrition, 51; acid and, 80–81; action list for, 146; amino acids in, 73–76, *75*; carbohydrates in, 74–75; diets for, 78–79; fats in, 71–72; gluten and, 81–82; immune system and, 33, 82–83, *84*; minerals in, 77–78; organic foods for, 128; pH levels and, *85*, 85–86; proper, 69–70; protein in, 72; to rebuild teeth, 84–85; summary of, 86–87; universe balance and, 128–29; vitamins and, 70, 78; water and, 70

Nutrition and Physical Degeneration, 13

obesity, 2, 49, 54

oil: good, 71–72; pulling, 36

Omega 3: fatty acids, *84*, test, 78

optimal health, achieve, 1, 7, 47, 67, 105, 142–45

optimal health plan: action list for, 146–47; dental, 145; free will, 146; God's law and, 146; love, 146; medical, 145; nutrition, 146; stress, 146; universal responsibility in, 146; world view in, 146

oral bacteria, diversity of, 13

oral health: chakras and, 98–99, *99*; downward causation and, *102*, 102–4, *103*; energy levels and, 96–97,

97; Kirlian photography and, 97–98, *98*; matter and energy affecting, 89–104, *92, 93, 95, 97, 98, 99, 102, 103*; meridian systems and, 100; physics and, 90–95, *92, 93, 95*; solutions for, 100–1
oral irrigator, 27–31, 38
oral lichen planus, 60
oral rinses, 37, 43
organic foods, 128
osteopathic physicians (DO), 66
oxidative stress, 49, 56; chronic inflammation and, 67, 108; dental toxicity and, 56; reduction of, 9
oxygen, 51, 60

para-aminobenzoic acid, 62
Parkinson's disease, 60
parotid gland, 20, *21*
PBDEs. *See* Polybrominated Diphenyl Ether
PCBs. *See* polychlorinated biphenyls
Peace, 5, 95
pellicle, 44
Perio Aid, instructions for, 35
periodontal gum therapies, 32
periodontal (gum) pockets, 22, *29*, 31–32, 34–35
periodontist, 46
periodontitis, 54. *See also* gum disease
pesticides, 122
pet delegates, 127–28
pH. *See* potential of Hydrogen
PHG. *See* Public Health Goal
phosphorous, 20, 43, 51, 77, 87; crystal, 15
physics: God's, *92*; Newtonian, 3, 90, *92*; quantum, 89, 91–92, *92*, 103, 137, 141; the world and, 90–91
plaque, 6; amyloid, 60; controlling, 18–23; dangerous, 32; dental, *16, 43*; non-specfic hypothses 18, 50; specific htpothses, 19, 50; quantity of, 18

play, 101, 126, 128
Polybrominated Diphenyl Ether (PBDEs), 122
Polychlorinated Biphenyls (PCBs), 122
positive thinking, 129–30
potential of Hydrogen (pH), 37, 39, 41, 65, 85–86
Pottenger, Dr., 13
Povidone iodine, 42
Prayer, 59, 94, 130, 140
Price, Weston, Dr., 13, 71, 79, 133
Prime One, 108
protein, in nutrition, 72
psychoimmunology, 110–11
pulp, of tooth, *29*, 51
pyridoxine supplement, 82–83

quantum physics, 89, 91–92, *92*, 103, 133, 137, 141

RBCs. *See* red blood cells
RCT (Root Canal Treatment), 4
red blood cells (RBCs), 53
reiki healing, 67
religions, traditional, 125
Rennou, 45
reproductive system, dysfunction of, 60
respiratory infections, 2, 49, 54
rest, 142
riboflavin, *84*
ripple effect, 123, 140–41
root canals, 50, 56; endodontic treatment for, *55*; meridian systems and, 100; studies of, 57; treated teeth, 61–62
rose oil, *118*

sacred spaces, 142
SAD. *See* Standard American Diet
saliva glands, 20, 43
saponification, 36
Scheinin, Arje, 40
scurvy, 53, 76
sealer cement, 57
Sears, Barry, Dr., 71

selenium, *84*
Sensodyne, 45
Septocaine, 62
serum albumin, 61
sesame oil, 36
Shrock, Dean, PhD, 121
Sigafoos, Gary, Dr., 34
sleep, 101, 126
Slots, Jorgen, Dr., 37
snacks, and soft drinks, 85
sodium fluoride, 64
sodium hypochlorite, 37
sodium monofluorophosphate, 64
soft picks, 35
specifically targeted antimicrobial
    peptide (STAMPs), 38
spiritual/energy model, 50, 51
spiritual frequencies, 138–39
spiritual healing, 133–34; blessings
    for, 130–31; chemistry and, 59–60;
    church and, 142; connections
    between, 141–42; energy levels and,
    138–39; fasting and, 142; forgiveness
    and, 123–24; indents and, 138–39;
    love and, 136; medication for, 142;
    prayer and intention for, 130; sacred
    spaces for, 142; spiritual frequencies
    and, 138–39; toolkit for, 139–40
spiritual toolkit, 139–43
spirochetes, 18–19
STAMPS. *See* specifically targeted
    antimicrobial peptide
Standard American Diet (SAD), 12, 72
stevia, 86
strep mutans, 14–15; lollipops and, 38
streptococcus, 18
stress: action list for, 146; anxiety
    from, 108; chronic inflammation
    and, 108; depression from, 108;
    effects of, 108; energy indents and,
    108; environmental, 107; indents
    and, 112–13, 138–39; jaw problems
    from, 108; negative, 120; oral,
    108–9; oxidative, 67, 108; psycho-
    immunological balance from, 108,

110–11; response to, 120; root causes
    of, 107; teeth grinding from, 108;
    TMJD and, 108, 111–12; tooth loss
    and, 109–10; victim mentality and,
    108, 113–16
strontium-chloride, 45, 82, *84*
sugar, and flour, 13, 20, 74–75, 80, 83,
    129
suicidal ideations, 60
sulfur, 60
supplements, for gum health, *84*
systemic theory, cavities, 19
Szent-Gyorgyi, Albert, 53

tablets, red-dissolving, 24
tartar, 13
teeth: anatomy of, *29*; extraction of, 9;
    gums and, 22–27; home care for,
    2, 22–27, 38; loss of, 108, 109–10;
    natural rebuilding of, 43–44; re-
    mineralization of, 45
teeth-body connection, *58*
teeth grinding, 108–10
temporomandibular joint disorder
    (TMJD), 111–12; from stress, 108
Tennant, Jerry, MD, 56
Tetrachloroethylene, 122
Theodent, 45
therapies, adjunctive, 43
thieves, 25–26

thyroiditis, 60
TMJD. *See* temporomandibular joint
    disorder
Toluene, 122
tooth. *See* teeth
tooth-body connection, 49, *52*
toothbrush, electric, 24, 27–28,
tooth brushing, 19; for acid attack, 26;
    amount of time, 24, 26–27; brush
    recommendation for, 24; for cavity
    protection, 26; ; sugar and, 26;
    tablets for, 24; technique for, 23–24,
    42; teeth health steps for, 22–28;
    toothpaste and, 25, 119

tooth decay, prevention of: arginine, 41, 73, 85; baking soda, 41, 43, 119; Dentiva, 39, 42, 46, 145; Loloz lollipops, 38, 42, 46, 145; MI Paste, 39, 42, 46, 145; Xylitol, 39–41, 43, 82–83, 122
tooth enamel, 15, *29*
toothpaste, *50*; apatite-forming, 45; baking soda in, 119; commercial, 25, 50; energy levels and, 118; essential oils and, 25–26, *118*; FDA and, 49; fluoride and, 117; homemade, 119–20; types of, 25–26
tooth picking, 33–35, *34*
toxins: chemical, 122; metals, 61, 101; reductions of, 9; release of, 60–61
treatments: fear-based, 3, *4*; patient-led, 33; refusal of, 33
triclosan, 65

ulcers, 61
universal responsibility, 146
universe balance: blessings for, 130–31; diet and nutrition for, 128–29; pet delegates for, 127–28; play as, 128; positive thinking and, 129–30; practical tools for, 127; prayer and intention for, 130; teeth and, 125–31
upward causation, *102*, 102–4

vegetables, 73–75
victimization, 113–16
victim mentality, 108, 113–16, 120–21, 126
vitamin A, *84*
vitamin C, 53–54, 76, 82–83, *84*
vitamin D, 54, 75, 76, 82, *84*
vitamin K, 82–83
vitamins, 76; deficiency of, 75, *75*; essential, 78; nutrition and, 70

water, 92, 114; environmental effects on, 94; life and, 137–38; nutrition and, 70
water crystals, 89, 92, *93*
Waterpik, *29,* 30
Wellness, 1, 20
white blood cells (WBCs), 53
Why Love Heals, 121
Wiener, Constance, PhD, 109
Work, 101, 126
Wright, Johnathan, M.D., 82–83

Xylitol, 39–43, 82–83, 122

Zero Point Field, 89
zinc, 60, 77, *84*
zirconia, 59
Zone diet, 71, 78, 146

About the Authors

Rev. Dr. Stephen A. Lawrence, a licensed dentist in California and an ordained mitred archpriest, has dedicated his career to helping people achieve and maintain optimal health and vitality. Over the course of his three-decade long professional life, he has earned degrees and certifications in theocentric healing, behavioral chiropathy, nutritional education, and religious counseling, which have led him to become one of America's leaders in the field of holistic dental health care, and spiritual and nutritional counseling. His purpose in life is to share his knowledge through lectures, courses, journals, and now books, all with the aim of helping patients, practitioners, and those searching for more meaningful and lasting pathways find better health, happiness, and peace.

David Tabatsky is a writer, editor, teacher, and performing artist. He is the co-author of *Reimagining Women's Cancers* and *Reimagining Men's Cancers*, author of *Write for Life: Communicating Your Way Through Cancer*, co-author of Chicken Soup for the Soul's *The Cancer Book: 101 Stories of Courage, Support and Love,* and editor of Elizabeth Bayer's *It's Just a Word*. He co-authored, with Bruce Kluger, *Dear President Obama: Letters of Hope from Children Across America*, *The Intelligent Divorce*, Books One and Two with Dr. Mark Banschick, and was the consulting editor for Marlo Thomas's *New York Times* bestseller, *The Right Words at the Right Time*, Volume 2: *Your Turn*. His memoir, *American Misfit*, was published in November 2017. Please visit www.tabatsky.com and www.writeforlife.info.

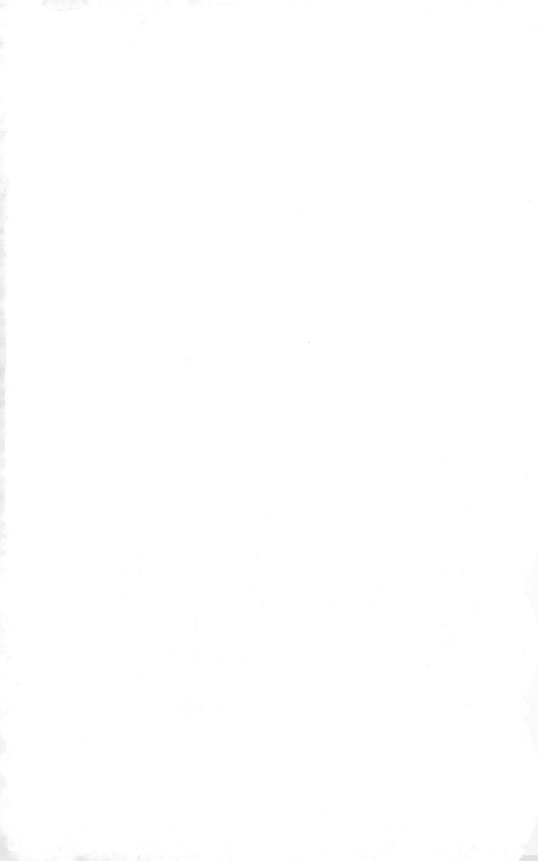